Eat to Beat the Flu

Eat to Beat the Flu

Prevent seasonal viruses with simple food choices

Jill Fleming, MS, RD

Inspiration Presentations Press
La Crosse, Wisconsin

For information, please contact:
Inspiration Presentations Press
P.O. Box 3372, La Crosse, WI 54602-3372
www.SimpleLifestyleChoices.com
Jill@SimpleLifestyleChoices.com

First printing 2010

ISBN 978-0-9754888-0-5

This book is dedicated to Nikolai, Brigette, and Peter.

All three of you have helped me learn how to become a patient mother, a great cook and a natural nurturer with food and lifestyle choices.
You are such a gift to me. Thank you.

AUTHOR'S NOTE

As with all natural health promotion programs, you should obtain your physician's permission and seek his or her supervision before and while you are following the advice provided in *Eat To Beat The Flu*. This is particularly important if you have a medical condition, such as cancer, diabetes, high blood pressure, heart disease or kidney disease. The author and publisher disclaim any liability arising directly or indirectly from the use of the *Eat To Beat The Flu* program.

CONTENTS

INTRODUCTION

It was October 29, 2009. I had just finished presenting a keynote address for 300 women at a Woman's Wellness Event in Pine Bluff, Arkansas. The title of the presentation was "Thin People Don't Clean Their Plates," which is my area of expertise, since this is also the title of my first book. At the end of my presentation, approximately 100 of the ladies rushed the stage with questions and to have their books signed.

When the last person left, I packed my bags and loaded my rental car. As I set off on the hour-long drive to the Little Rock airport, I was feeling really good. I celebrated by singing loudly to a couple of great songs. After several miles had passed, I began to hear that nagging question in the back of my head, "Am I making a big enough difference in the world?"

I had heard this question several times during my 18 year career as a registered dietitian. When I was a clinical dietitian and only saw one patient at a time, I wanted to help more people. I then created and taught weight loss programs for two different hospitals and fitness centers. I was then able to help 15 to 25 people reach their weight loss goals at one time, but I still felt I could make a bigger difference.

Then I joined the National Speaker Association and learned how to give keynote presentations to large audiences. My audiences are now anywhere from 50 to 2,000 people at one time, but I was again feeling like there was something more I could do, but I didn't know what that was. Since my career expertise is as a weight loss dietitian, I knew I needed to stay true to my non-diet approach to optimal health message.

One of my favorite cartoons is of two women standing over a coffin talking. One says, "They say diet pills caused her heart problems..." and the other lady replies, "Yeah, but doesn't she look great in a size 7?" This is a cartoon I love to share with my weight loss classes and audiences as we discuss the real reason for weight loss, which isn't to just look good in your "skinny jeans."

Making better lifestyle choices to reach your optimal weight is great, but achieving your optimal health and energy level is truly the goal. If you don't have your health, you don't have anything. When you lose weight by making simple lifestyle choices, you will decrease your risk of chronic diseases and substantially increase your energy level.

So I got to the Little Rock airport. After I returned the rental car, made it through security and got redressed after being frisked in security, I called home to check-in. My husband said Peter, our seven year old son didn't eat anything for lunch, which is unusual for him. He said he hoped he wasn't getting sick.

Many of our friends had kids sick with the flu. H1N1 is the current flu strain everyone is afraid of contracting. As a gentle reminder, I said, "Please be sure to feed all three kids a big salad, with carrots at dinner tonight." Being a Registered Dietitian, I was always using food and it's almost magical properties to keep our family healthy.

My husband replied, “About that... I have bad news.” You know that kid in Peter’s tennis class, Jesse? He died last night. He had pneumonia.” I felt sick. Then I felt sad for his mother, thinking that Jesse could just as easily have been my seven year old! Then a strange thought came to me; I wondered if I could have done anything to help prevent Jesse’s death.

It was at that exact moment that I knew... I needed to share my knowledge of nutrition and how food can prevent the viruses and bacteria that are stealing our children from us. Children are being robbed of their precious lives needlessly.

This was a message to me, from God, that I need to speak up and speak out against seasonal viruses. It would be selfish of me not to. The tiny voice inside of myself, trying to protect me, saying I would set myself up for public scrutiny from those who disagreed with my opinion was quieted. Who cares if I have to withstand the criticism from those who are only out for their own personal gain with a product or a program to sell?

A few days later, shortly after Halloween, I was walking Peter to his second grade classroom when his teacher came running down the hall toward us with a frantic look on her face. She said, “I need to warn you! We had eight kids from our classroom out sick yesterday, two of them vomited in the classroom before they left and one of them was sitting right next to Peter. We are Lysoling every surface every night. We don’t know what else to do!”

Over the course of the next week, 15 of the 16 kids in Peter’s class were out sick, including his teacher! Peter was the only child from his classroom who didn’t get sick. We have three children who attend three different schools. Despite the fact that they have exposure to so many children and viruses, not one of our children got sick this year, other than the occasional runny nose.

This is the third year in a row, since I've been paying attention, that our entire family has not had more than a slight cold. No one has had the flu. I decided to take a look at our family's daily lifestyle choices and work backward to find the research that would reveal why we were not getting sick despite having the same exposure to viruses as others.

After digging into the research, I discovered that the virus-preventing lifestyle choices our family was making all fit neatly into one of three categories. They are:

1. **Alkalinize and oxygenate your body.**
2. **Strengthen your immune and lymphatic systems.**
3. **Prevent viruses from entering your body.**

This book will provide you with the simple lifestyle choices to prevent seasonal viruses, as well as the research behind these recommendations.

The exciting news is that while you are probably reading this book to save yourself and your children from a premature death as a result of a seasonal virus, most of the recommendations in this book are consistent with my weight loss research strategies. Therefore, following the *Eat To Beat The Flu* strategies will also help you shed excess body fat, as you begin to nourish and respect the amazing temple your body truly is.

I will never know if the information contained in this book could have saved Jesse's life. I can only wonder and be sad I did not get this information out sooner. My hope is that after reading this book, you will share this potentially, lifesaving information with your own family, friends, neighbors and even strangers.

CHAPTER 1

The Wellness Triangle

Your present circumstances don't determine where you can go; they merely determine where you start.

—Nido Quebin

The basic foundation for optimal health is simply a matter of balancing your daily lifestyle choices.

The Wellness Triangle is a simple foundation that I created in 1993 to represent the three areas of your lifestyle choices that all need to be balanced. I originally made this model for my *Thin Choices* weight loss clients to teach them the importance of achieving balance in all of their daily lifestyle choices.

The Wellness Triangle, shown on the next page, represents the ultimate balance for optimal health in a person's life. When aspiring to reach optimal health, each corner of the triangle needs to be in balance with the other two corners. If you pay attention to all three areas, you will achieve your health improvement goals.

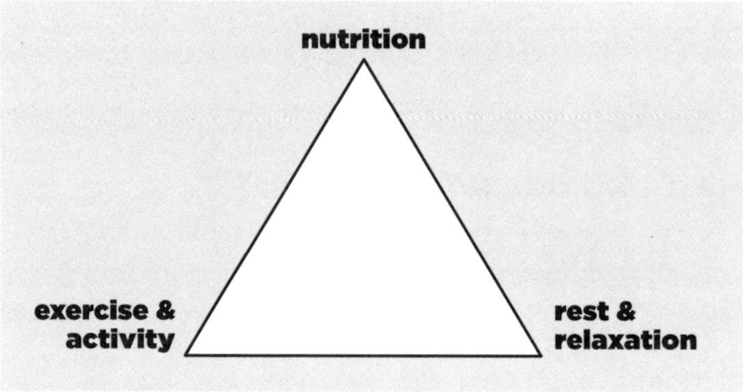

Nutrition corner

Ideally, paying attention to the nutrition corner means that you are feeding your body real, healthy foods in small quantities throughout the day. This corner also includes a good intake of water, with limited caffeine and alcohol consumption. You are listening to your body for clues and not over or under feeding it.

You will learn more about specific foods to eat or omit throughout the remainder of this book. The food and beverage choices you make each day can protect you against viruses and disease or increase your risk of becoming sick and dying prematurely.

Exercise corner

The exercise corner is in its ideal state when you are participating in an aerobic activity, moving your body a minimum of 30 minutes most days of the week. Aerobic exercise helps your body take in extra oxygen, which helps oxygenate your body. The specific types of exercises that are most beneficial to improve the function of your lymphatic system are discussed in chapter 13.

Lifting weights or participating in toning exercises a few

times each week also enhances your exercise corner of the wellness triangle. Being an active person is a bonus, as this will also help keep your lymphatic system pumping.

Rest and relaxation corner

The rest and relaxation corner of the wellness triangle is optimal when you sleep an average of seven to eight hours each night. This suggested amount of sleep time is backed up by recent research that revealed most individuals who slept for this amount of time woke up feeling refreshed and alert. Sleeping more than eight hours per night was not recommended by this research.

Some individuals may find that they do not need this much sleep each night, whereas others will feel that they need more. Gauge how much sleep you personally need on how you feel upon waking. Keep a sleep journal for a week. Write down how much sleep you got each night versus how you felt the next morning. Lack of sleep causes stress to the body and disrupts hormone levels within your body.

This sleep, in a perfect world, is not restless, but sound and without interruptions. If you are overweight, you may find that you do not sleep in the perfect world. With excess weight, you may experience back aches or muscle cramps. Many individuals who are overweight will also experience sleep apnea. These problems will lessen with weight loss.

The second half of the rest and relaxation corner of the wellness triangle is relaxing or stress-reduction. Stress, which seems to be a normal state for most Americans, causes an imbalance in the R&R corner. Stress will disrupt sleep, change eating habits and hormones. If stress is not controlled, your body will be more vulnerable to viruses and other preventable diseases. Deep breathing and meditation are two excellent methods used to relax your mind and body. Both will be discussed in more detail in Chapter 12.

Balance your triangle

If you neglect any one corner of the triangle, the triangle is out of balance and you are not in optimal health. For example, if you are not getting enough sleep to awake feeling refreshed and alert, you will have an increased appetite, causing you to eat more junk, processed, and refined foods. When you eat poorly, in addition to not having enough sleep, you will rarely have the energy to move your body or engage in exercise.

If you increase caffeine to compensate for the lack of sleep, the whole triangle is out of balance. Because of the caffeine, you will most likely not experience a good night's sleep the next night either. Consequently, the cycle of eating poorly and not exercising continues.

To break this vicious cycle, you must balance the three corners of your wellness triangle. To begin, exercise for at least 30 minutes to make your body physically tired. This will help you get a better night's sleep. After a good night's sleep, you will be able to control your appetite and improve your whole triangle.

I was recently teaching a healthy living class for women over the age of 50 at our local YMCA. Ten of the participants complained they no longer get enough quality sleep. They said they are often tired during the day, yet have a hard time sleeping at night. After just three weeks of adding aerobic exercise (three times per week) and improving their nutrition choices, all 10 women now say they are sleeping better than they have in years.

The nutrition changes they made were to limit caffeine, alcohol and sugar as they increased their intake of fruit, vegetables and water. With these few simple lifestyle changes, they are sleeping better, have less stress and have balanced their entire Wellness Triangles.

A near-perfect scenario is that you sleep peacefully for seven to eight hours at night. You wake up refreshed and go for a morning walk outside for at least 30 minutes. You then eat a balanced diet full of fruit and vegetables, lean protein and whole grains, drink plenty of water and limit both caffeinated and alcoholic beverages. You dedicate a minimum of seven minutes to meditation or deep breathing daily, where you quiet your mind. At the end of the day, you go to bed feeling tired and get another restful night of sleep, going on to repeat this cycle the next day.

It may seem as if I am overly simplifying the process to reach optimal health. It truly is this simple. It is not always easy in the real world, but the longer you live this simplified approach to wellness, the easier it will become.

CHAPTER 2

The pH Scale

To acquire balance means to achieve that happy medium between the minimum and the maximum that represents your optimum. The minimum is the least you can get by with. The maximum is the most you're capable of. The optimum is the amount or degree of anything that is most favorable toward the ends you desire.

—*Nido Quebin*

pH = potential Hydrogen

acid **neutral** **alkaline**

0 1 2 3 4 5 6 7 8 9 10 11 12 13 14

Remember learning about the pH scale in high school chemistry class? We learned that a pH of 7 is neutral, 0 up to 7 is acidic, and greater than 7 is alkaline or a base? Turning liquids in the beaker from red to blue with just a few drops of solution was fun, but it didn't really mean a whole lot in terms of real life.

Well, it turns out that our bodies operate best with a pH of

7.4, which is slightly alkaline. When you are in optimal health, this will be the pH of your blood, spinal fluid, urine and saliva.

Simple saliva or urine pH test to determine your body's environment

Measuring the pH of your saliva or urine is an easy way to check your susceptibility to seasonal viruses, such as a cold or the flu. Ideally, your saliva or urine should be at a PH of 7.4, or slightly alkaline.

You can easily check the pH of your saliva or urine for a quick look at the pH of your body's fluids using a strip of litmus paper. You will want to purchase a package of litmus paper test strips. You can find these at your local pharmacy. Since the pH of your saliva and urine will be more variable, due to your recent diet, emotions, etc., having the pH of your blood checked at your next doctor appointment would be the ideal test to determine your blood's pH level.

To be sure you are getting the best, most accurate saliva reading, you will want to get your saliva's pH reading in the morning before you have had anything to eat or drink. You should collect saliva in your mouth and swallow it. Do this a second time to be sure your saliva is clean.

The third time you fill your mouth with saliva, spit onto the testing square of the PH test strip. Compare the color of your test strip's square with the color chart on the package. Your goal is for your saliva to turn neutral or slightly alkaline. This may be the green or the blue color, depending on which test strips your purchase.

If your saliva is acidic (below 7), it will most likely be yellow. You will want to test it again, but be sure to wait at least two hours after eating or drinking anything.

The saliva pH parallels the extra cellular fluid of the body.

The saliva pH of a healthy person is in the 7.1 to 7.5, slightly alkaline range. Most children will have a saliva pH of 7.5. Many adults will have a pH of 6.5 or lower, which could be due to a calcium deficiency of aging or daily lifestyle choices.

Checking your urine is also easy. You will want to urinate on the small square of the pH test strip for just one-second. Ideally, this will not be your first urine of the morning, as urine pH is more acidic in the morning. Keep in mind that a midday reading may be influenced by the acid or alkaline forming potential of the foods and beverages you have consumed.

Acidosis

If you have ever heard of acidosis, you are probably familiar with keto-acidosis (related to diabetes or consuming a high protein diet), or lactic acidosis (a result of over-exercising) or renal acidosis (associated with kidney failure). What we are talking about in relation to your diet and lifestyle choices is metabolic acidosis. Metabolic acidosis is a pH imbalance in which the body has accumulated too much acid and does not have enough bicarbonate to effectively neutralize the effects of the acid.

When you are in an acidic state, your body has an excess of H+ (hydrogen) ions. When you are in a healthy, slightly alkaline state, you have an excess of OH- (hydroxyl) ions. Excess hydroxyl ions can combine to form water and the excess oxygen is then available to oxygenate your body's tissues.

CHAPTER 3

Theories of Disease

Develop success from failures. Discouragement and failure are two of the surest stepping stones to success.

—Dale Carnagie

Should we try to kill all the flies or clean up the garbage attracting them?

Louis Pasteur

In the 1800's, Louis Pasteur, the inventor of pasteurization, developed the single-formed (monomorphic) germ theory. This theory states that there are fixed, external germs (microbes) which invade the body and cause a variety of diseases. These diseases include everything from pneumonia to cancer.

To get well, you must identify and then kill whatever germ made you sick. Usually drugs, surgery, radiation and chemotherapy are recommended. Prevention includes vaccines and sometimes drugs.

Claude Bernard

Around the same time that Pasteur was doing his research, another scientist, Claude Bernard came up with the theory that the body's ability to heal itself was dependent on its general health or internal environment. Thus, disease occurred only when the terrain or internal environment of the body became favorable to disease.

Antoine Bechamp

Then comes Antoine Bechamp. He is a medical doctor and a university professor who has degrees in chemistry, biology and physics. He built upon and extended Bernard's work, developing his own theory of health and disease, which revolved around the concept of pleomorphism (meaning "many-formed").

Bechamp discovered tiny organisms or microorganisms that could take on many forms, depending on the condition of the host or biological terrain. He called them microzymas. He found these microzymas to be present in all things, living and dead.

His theory states that disease results when microzyma change form, functions and toxicity based on the host. Bad bacteria, viruses and fungi are the forms assumed when the terrain favors disease. These "bad microzyma" give off toxic byproducts, further weakening the terrain.

This makes me think about the rotting log in the woods. When I turn it over, the fungi growing on it is working to decompose the wood. Where did the fungi come from? Why doesn't it decompose the healthy, living trees?

Who is right?

There is documentation stating that toward the end of Pasteur's life, he admitted Bernard and Bechamp were right about the terrain being important in the prevention of disease. If you believe the external germ is the enemy that needs to be killed once it invades the body, then there is nothing you can do to prevent seasonal viruses, other than get your influenza vaccines every year.

Since our family of five has been virus-free for over three years, except for a few sniffles, without the potential protection of influenza vaccines, I strongly support the pleomorphic theory of disease. I am confident we can prevent viruses, bacteria and fungi from invading our bodies and making us sick by making a few simple lifestyle choices on a regular basis.

Many of my weight loss clients have also reported being more resistant to colds and the flu since they started making better lifestyle choices. Once they balanced their Wellness Triangle, they experienced fewer bacteria and virus related illnesses.

People mingling: Schools and travel

Louis Pasteur's germ theory is based on the idea that germs are the enemy and we should avoid contact with sick people at all costs. We have all been told to wash our hands frequently and to only sneeze into our elbows. We are all walking around with antibacterial gels and avoiding the customary handshake.

When our kids ride the school bus, attend classes and play with their friends at recess, we cringe at the thought of them being so vulnerable. Every time you board an airplane, you are taking a chance that someone around you is sick. The reality is that you are increasing your risk of exposure every time you are in a social setting or traveling.

Does this mean you need to home-school your children and stay home during the cold and flu months? Of course not! The real key is to create an environment in our bodies that is a poor host environment for viruses. While there are a few specific strategies you can use when you are traveling (discussed in chapter 14) to stay healthy, how you fuel, move and rest your body daily are the most important habits.

CHAPTER 4

Your Body Wants Balance

Let thy food be thine medicine.

—Hippocrates

Your lungs, kidneys, skeleton and muscles all work together to keep your body in optimum pH balance, or slightly alkaline. Your body truly wants to be balanced and healthy.

Role of your lungs

Something as natural as breathing is helping keep your body in proper pH balance. As you breathe in oxygen, you are oxygenating your body tissues. As you exhale carbon dioxide, which is acidic, you are alkalinizing your body. Making a point to breathe deeply throughout the day will help naturally decrease your body's acidity.

Your kidneys, skeleton, and osteoporosis

Your kidneys have two very important jobs. One is to maintain the proper fluid balance in your body. The other is to keep your body fluids slightly alkaline, with a pH of approximately

7.4. When your body is operating more acidic, your kidneys will take buffering minerals from your bones. These minerals are Calcium and magnesium. Unfortunately, since these minerals are needed to keep your bones strong, you will be increasing your chance of getting osteoporosis and other bone related diseases.

A study published in *The Journal of Nutrition* in 2008 conducted a one-month dietary intervention with 23- to 76-year-old men and women. This study showed that a diet high in bicarbonate (high fruits and vegetables) and potassium significantly reduced bone turnover. Longer-term studies will need to be conducted.

Your muscles and Restless Leg Syndrome (RLS)

Another buffering mineral is potassium. When your body is acidic, your kidneys will take potassium, as well as calcium and magnesium from your muscles. It is interesting to note that calcium, magnesium and potassium all have an effect on muscle contractions, relaxations and nerve transmission.

The combined deficiency of these three minerals could be responsible for the annoying jumpiness of Restless Leg Syndrome (RLS). A lack of calcium, magnesium and potassium can make the large muscles in the legs hyperirritable. Could it be our overly acidic diets and lifestyles that are causing a deficiency of these three minerals in our bodies?

Only recently has medical science even recognized RLS as a big problem. According to a Harvard Health Publication, most surveys peg the prevalence of Restless Leg Syndrome at approximately 10 percent of the population of the United States. The intensity of RLS ranges from mild to moderate to severe.

A few weeks ago, I was visiting my parents at their house and my dad was sitting on the couch reading the paper. All of a sudden, he jumped up; almost as if a flea had bitten him. He threw down the paper, quickly went to the kitchen, peeled a banana and took a big bite of it. I started to laugh. I said, "What was that? You suddenly realized you were hungry for a banana?" He said, "No, my leg jumped! That means I need some potassium for my Restless Leg Syndrome, so I am eating a banana."

Could it be that his body is acidic and he is losing calcium, magnesium and potassium from his muscles as his kidneys work to buffer the acidity? Maybe. By the way, he also suffers from gout.

CHAPTER 5

The Standard American Diet and Lifestyle

We are living in a world today where lemonade is made from artificial flavors and furniture polish is made from real lemons.

—Alfred E. Newman

Americans are overfed and undernourished

With two-thirds of Americans classified as overweight and one-third as obese, you would never guess that most overweight people are actually undernourished. How does this happen? With the Standard American Diet, also known appropriately as S.A.D., we are consuming and excess of processed and sugary foods.

The Standard American Diet is:

- *High in calories*
- *High in animal fats*
- *High in unhealthy fats: saturated, hydrogenated, trans fats*

- *High in sugar and corn syrup*
- *Low in fiber*
- *High in processed foods*
- *Low in complex carbohydrates*
- *Low in plant-based foods, especially fruits and vegetables*

Americans following this typical Standard American Diet feel as if they are always hungry, because the cells of their body have not been fed. Their cells will request more food and will receive additional nutrient-stripped food that does not satisfy their requirement for optimal function. Excess calories are stored as fat and the cycle continues.

The scale continues to rise. The incidence of cancer, coronary artery disease (CAD) and potentially life-threatening viruses increases. We do not need better health care at this point, we just need to nourish our bodies better. We need to switch from the focus of quantity to the focus on quality.

When the reports from the Centers for Disease Control (CDC) first came out revealing that those aged 5 to 24 have the highest risk of infection rate and those ages 25 to 49 have the highest death rates from the H1N1 flu, I was not surprised. This is because after doing thousands of food intake interviews, these are the groups following the S.A.D. way of eating.

The researchers even commented that those over 64 years of age seem to have some kind of immunity to the virus. My work as a Registered Dietitian has revealed to me that those over 64 years of age tend to eat the most vegetables and real food. I define real food as food that comes from nature, in it's own packaging and grew with sun and rain or water.

When I am speaking to elementary students, they like the term "grow food" in reference to "real food." They understand that food that has grown with sun and rain or water will help their bodies grow. You may be surprised to learn that many of the students I have presented nutrition topics to do like many fruits and vegetables, but state that their parents just don't buy them or prepare them very often.

Americans are crazy-busy

We are all living in such a fast-paced society, that we don't have time to take care of ourselves anymore. You work all day, fill your evenings with meetings and sporting events or activities for your kids. I've often heard individuals refer to life as "crazy-busy". It is as if being "crazy-busy" is a badge of honor. The person who appears the busiest wins the prize!

Is your health suffering because of this hectic, over-scheduled lifestyle? Are you really getting ahead or are you just racing to your grave? When it comes to your health, you need to put yourself back on the top of your "to do" list. You shouldn't have to squeeze exercise in between events. You don't have to accept the fact that you eat while sitting in the driver's seat of your car, more often than at your dining room table, as normal.

The 3 F's to limit or avoid

When I was conducting the research for my first book, *Thin People Don't Clean Their Plates*, I discovered the majority of thin people avoided, what I call the three F's: fast food, fried food and fake food. While many of them did occasionally eat these foods, they were not a regular part of their diets. They cited reasons such as not feeling well after consuming these types of foods and wanting to set a good example for others, such as children, as reasons for avoiding these choices.

This is interesting, as these same types of foods should be avoided to improve the over-all quality of your diet to prevent the invasion of your body by seasonal viruses. Fast food, fried food and fake food all have been either mechanically or chemically altered and processed to make them taste better. The more processed your food choice is, the fewer health benefits it will offer to your body.

When choosing a food choice that is fried or processed or junk, consider it a "treat" for your mouth. Eat the smallest amount you need to feel satisfied and then move on. Eating like this is in contrast to how most American's approach unhealthy eating choices, which is with the all-or-nothing mentality. They feast on the junky food, promising themselves that they will eat better tomorrow ... or Monday!

Too busy to cook

Many busy Americans complain they are too busy to cook and sit down for family meals. Their kids are over-scheduled and they are rushing home from work and off to the next sporting event. Going through the nearest drive through to grab some burgers, fries and sugary sodas is all too common. The key to finding the time to cook is to plan ahead and know your menu in advance.

To avoid eating on impulse, you will want to make a basic rotating menu plan. Since most families rotate the same six to eight meals through their house each month, you will find that establishing the menu plan based on your family's preferences will be easy. Your family will not get bored with the meals and it will help simplify your planning and cooking schedule.

You don't need to get too specific with your menu. You only need to plan the main food category plus a vegetable for each meal in a week. Since the evening meal is the meal that most people tend to struggle with, this will be the meal you should be planning. Here is an example of our family's basic meal plan for supper:

Monday	*Italian or "pasta night" + salad*
Tuesday	*Mexican or "taco Tuesday"*
Wednesday	*Crock-pot cooking (great for busy sports nights)*
Thursday	*Leftovers or sandwiches*
Friday	*Pizza night + garden salad*
Saturday	*Seafood Saturday*
Sunday	*Soup and salad night*

Once you have your basic menu pattern for the week, you will need to get the ingredients needed for each meal. Read through the recipes you plan to make for the week and create your shopping list from these ingredients. Keep staples, such as tomato sauce and multigrain pasta available for nights when you don't have much time to prepare the meal.

Be sure to have plenty of fruit and vegetables available to add a big salad and some fresh or frozen fruit to each meal. On "taco Tuesday" you may decide to have diced tomatoes and chopped lettuce as your vegetable. Cucumber slices and carrot sticks are great sides for leftover or sandwich night. Mix up the vegetables so that you don't get bored, but alway have the salad bowl available for a back up with picky eaters.

It's not just about what you *are* eating...

It is often more about what your *are not* eating than what you *are* eating. Which food groups are lacking or missing from your current diet? For most Americans they will quickly identify that they are not consuming enough vegetables OR fruit. This is a great place to begin to improve your eating habits.

As you start to fuel your body with more nutritious foods, your cravings for sweets and junk food will almost disappear. You will finally feel in-control of your food choices, instead of the food controlling you. You will be amazed to notice that your body soon begins to crave healthier food choices.

The next time you are craving some chocolate or candy, eat an orange and then ask yourself if you still want the sweets. You will be amazed to notice that you will be satisfied with the naturally sweet orange. Many times you will even want to have another orange.

The reason you may not have been successful making positive changes to your diet in the past, is that the changes you have made were too restrictive. As soon as you know you can't eat pizza, all you can think about it pizza. When you are told you can't eat chocolate, you begin to obsess about it.

The best part about the Eat to Beat the Flu strategies, is that you *can* eat your favorite foods. In fact, you are encouraged to eat some of your favorite foods everyday! If your new eating plan is not individualized for you, you will not be able to make these healthier eating habits a permanent part of your life.

Lifestyle change program

To make these healthy eating and living strategies work for you and your family, you will need to individualize your diet. Keep in mind, that we are talking about what you eat on a daily basis, not a restrictive *diet*. Don't aim to have a perfect diet, instead focus on adding more quality foods to your menu and being "pretty good" most of the time.

Instead of working against your body, you are going to learn how to listen to it and give it what it needs to enable you to achieve your optimal health. Note that your body will begin to crave more of the foods that you feed it. Your body does crave optimal health.

Your attitude will determine your success. You need to realize that you alone are responsible for the foods you choose to put into your body. You need to quit blaming others for your poor health and start taking responsibility. How you choose to fuel your body during the cold and flu season will ultimately determine if and how severe of a case of the seasonal viruses you may get.

Remember when...

Remember when you used to eat at your grandparent's house or even your own house when you were a child? You always sat down as a family around the dining table. Meals were planned to include the four basic food groups, so they always included vegetables. A prayer of thanks was usually given for the food and good company. Meal time was relaxed and took almost an hour to serve and eat. Even doing the dishes was a family affair.

Families today have lost the bonding time meals together offer. We are in such a rush to make and eat the meal, we forget to slow down and really enjoy the food and companionship. The nutritional content of the meal is often compromised as we grab a fast meal or toss a frozen meal into the microwave.

When the reporters from the news stations were reporting H1N1 as a "young person's disease," no one seemed to make the connection that older people still tend to eat their vegetables and fruit with balanced meals. They are also more likely to sit down at a dining table instead of standing over the kitchen sink or eating off their lap in the car. Interesting...

Make your family's meal plan, shop for the groceries and plan to sit down together at the dining table for meals together most days of the week. Not only will the nutritional content of your family's dinner improve, but you will be amazed at how much your kids really do want to have your undivided attention. This is a great time to find out what is going on in your children's lives.

CHAPTER 6

Alkalinize and Oxygenate Your Body

Nothing would be more tiresome than eating and drinking if God had not made them a pleasure as well as a necessity.

—Voltaire

Viruses cannot exist in an alkaline, oxygen-rich environment

Cold and flu viruses need an acidic environment that lacks oxygen to live. When your diet consists of many processed, refined and sweet foods you are creating this ideal environment. No wonder so many kids get sick right after Halloween and Christmas!

Do you read the ingredient list on all of your food and beverage labels before your buy them? If a second grader can't pronounce the entire list of ingredients on the food label, you are probably consuming too many processed foods and chemicals. These processed and refined foods and beverages increase the acidity of your body fluids. The goal is to get back to eating *real* food and making *water* your primary choice of a beverage.

Junk foods, processed foods and fried foods all deplete oxygen stores. They use up more oxygen than they give off. Not to say you can't ever eat these foods, but if you do, you should make sure you are also taking in plenty of oxygen-rich plant-based foods that can help replace the lost oxygen.

Plant-based diet

Eating a plant-based diet, loaded with vegetables and fruit, is the best way to create an alkaline environment in your body. This doesn't necessarily mean you should follow a vegetarian diet. It means limiting the amount of animal products that you eat, turning to other sources of protein, and building meals around vegetables, fruit and healthy grains. It also means limiting your intake of processed, refined and preserved foods.

Over the past two decades, I have discovered that most Americans are much more successful in making dietary improvements when they focus on what they should *add* to their diet, instead of focusing on what they should *avoid*. When you begin to add more of the foods that nourish your body, you will naturally begin to cut back on the less healthy choices without feeling deprived. Since your body craves what you feed it, you will soon have an increased desire for those foods that nourish, oxygenate, alkalinize and energize your body.

"Five-A-Day" for better health

You may remember hearing about the five-a-day campaign to increase the consumption of fruit and vegetables by Americans to a total of five servings per day. This campaign was initiated by the Centers for Disease Control (CDC) and the Produce for Better Health Foundation (PBH) in 1991. Since the importance of fruit and vegetable consumption is so widely recognized due to repeated research studies, the campaign was then changed to the five-to-nine per day campaign. They have since partnered with many other organizations to launch a new public health initiative called "Fruits & Veggies—More Matters."

Consuming fruits and vegetables has been found to decrease your risk of cancer, heart disease, stoke and diabetes. Most Americans are aware of how beneficial fruit and vegetables are to their health, yet intake remains low. The most recent National Health and Nutrition Examination Survey (NHANES) data reveals an average intake of two and one-half servings of fruit or vegetables per day with only 20 percent of all Americans achieving the five per day goal.

Three reasons to consume more fruit or vegetables daily are to create an alkaline environment in your body fluids, to decrease your risk of preventable diseases and to lose weight. These foods have very few calories, are high in fiber, full of water and loaded in antioxidants and phytonutrients.

The word phytonutrient is a term coined to describe plant chemicals, with "phyto" meaning plant-based. You may already be aware of some phytonutrients, such as lycopene, which makes tomatoes red; lutein, the color of corn; beta-carotene, which makes carrots orange; chlorophyll, found in the leafy vegetables; and anthocyanin, giving the reds and blues to berries and grapes.

Many of the colored phytonutrients have structures that make them good antioxidants and therefore neutralize free radicals, to prevent cancer. Even the unpigmented vegetables, such as garlic and white onions contain important protective phytonutrients. Research is beginning to show the effects of phytonutrients on preventing cancer growth, hormone function, decreasing inflammation and improving immune and blood vessel function. All of these health improving qualities are found to be independent of their antioxidant nature.

While current intake of vegetables and fruit remains low, I am optimistic that we can more than double these numbers with a little planning. Despite the current USDA recommendation to consume five to nine servings of fruit or vegetables, I always recommend an intake of eight to ten servings daily for my weight loss clients and those who are interested in flu or cancer prevention. This may initially seem like a lot of fruit and vegetables, but with a little advanced preparation, it is a simple goal to achieve.

To make achieving this goal easier, I instruct my weight loss clients to consume one smoothie and one large salad daily. This will get you to your goal intake of eight to ten servings of fruit or vegetables daily. Believe it or not, this large amount of fruit and vegetables will only total roughly 400 calories per day or the number of calories in a large muffin.

The recommendation for how many servings of fruit and vegetables children should eat is less than that for adults, as their bodies are smaller. Your goal should be to help them consume a total of three to five one-half cup servings daily. The reason I say "help them" is because, as an adult, you will be responsible for the purchasing and preparing of the fruit and vegetables.

You will find that you do need to make more frequent trips to the grocery store or farmer's market to replenish your fruit bowl and produce section of your refrigerator. Our family of five goes through 35 bananas and up to five pounds of carrots each week!

Both fruit and vegetables help create an alkaline, oxygen-rich environment in your body. Viruses cannot live in this environment. Adults need to eat a minimum of three to five vegetables and two to four servings of fruit. Kids should be eating at least two to three (one-half cup each) servings of vegetables daily and two (tennis ball sized) servings of fruit per day.

Cut up vegetables and leave them sitting out for kids to snack on after school or before dinner. Include a salad with every dinner meal. Throw some shredded carrots and chopped apples into the muffins. Add some pumpkin to your pancakes.

Throw a handful of fresh spinach into the smoothie. Don't assume your kids won't eat their vegetables. My kids now ask for salads and carrots with lunch and dinner. Make it a general rule that each meal needs to include at least one or two fruits or vegetables and you will help kids easily reach their intake goal. Remember to be a good role model, as kids are watching you and want to do what you are doing.

Beneficial raw foods

Professor Paul Talalay, of the Johns Hopkins Medical School says, "The best and most widely recognized protection against cancer is the consumption of large quantities of vegetables, in particular crucifers like broccoli and broccoli sprouts which are very rich in chemicals that raise enzymes that destroy cancer causing chemicals."

All fruits and vegetables are good for you, but it is always best to include a variety in your diet. Plan to eat all of the colors of the rainbow everyday, as like colors tend to contain similar phytonutrients and benefits to your body.

Red *apples, cherries, raspberries, red bell peppers, strawberries and tomatoes.*

Orange *apricots, cantaloupe, carrots, mangos, oranges, peaches, pumpkins and sweet potatoes.*
Yellow *bananas, corn, grapefruit, lemons, pineapple, squash and yellow bell peppers.*
Green *avocado, basil, beans, cabbage, celery, green beans, green peppers, kale, lettuce, limes, parsley, pears, spinach and zucchini.*
Purple *beets, blackberries, blueberries, currants, eggplant, and red cabbage.*
White *cauliflower, garlic, onions and potatoes.*

Enzymes

There are two type of enzymes. They are digestive enzymes and metabolic enzymes. You naturally have metabolic enzymes in your body. These are the enzymes that help rejuvenate and repair cells in your body. You have a finite number and they cannot be replenish once they are gone.

Raw fruits, vegetables and a handful of other living foods, naturally contain digestive enzymes which help break your food down into a usable form of energy for your body. Enzymes help you digest your food. Since enzymes are proteins, they have a very specific three-dimensional structure. Unfortunately, once they are heated above 118 degrees, this structure can change and the enzymes are no longer able to assist with the digestion.

The process for digestion of cooked food demands much more energy than the digestion of raw food, since any naturally occurring enzymes have been destroyed. Instead of having digestive enzymes available to assist with digestion, your body will have to use metabolic enzymes to do this job. This is not to say that you should never eat cooked foods, it is just a good reminder that it is important to include plenty of raw fruits, vegetables and nuts daily. A great goal to strive for is to eventually consume a total of 50 percent (volume) of your food raw.

Raw nuts

Raw nuts, such as Brazil nuts and almonds, are a good source of heart healthy fats and protein. Raw nuts can counteract the benefits of the digestive enzymes because they contain enzyme inhibitors. To deactivate these inhibitors, you will want to soak your nuts in water overnight. Rinse them off in the morning, dry them with a towel and enjoy. You will find that the nuts plump up and actually taste better, plus are easier for your body to digest.

Nuts are a great source of the trace nutrient selenium, which is a cancer preventing antioxidant. One Brazil nut contains 100 percent of the recommended daily allowance for selenium. Researchers at the Unviersity of North Carolina discovered that influenza virus that has been passed through mice deficient in selenium, mutates and emerges from the mice more virulent than before.

In this study, they fed groups of mice either selenium-deficient or normal diets. Later, they exposed both groups to a mild strain of human influenza A. Rodents consuming too little selenium developed significantly more harmful lung inflammation, which also lasted considerable longer, than mice that developed the flu but had normal diets. The conclusion is that something similar happens in humans who are deficient in selenium, since humans and mice are so biologically similar.

Another study demonstrated that a human virus normally harmless to mice mutates and becomes more dangerous after infecting selenium-deficient and vitamin E deficient mice. Following mutation, the virus can then infect and damage the hearts of mice with no selenium deficiency. One of the researchers, Orville Levander stated, "The fact that we're now seeing 29 mutations in this one segment of the genome of influenza virus just as a result of nutritional manipulation to me is just extraordinary."

Specific raw foods

Carrots

Carrots are an excellent source of antioxidant compounds and the richest vegetable source of the pro-vitamin A carotenes. The antioxidant compounds in carrots help protect against cardiovascular disease, cancer and also promote good vision, especially night vision. Eating as little as one large carrot per day can help improve your vision, decrease your risk of cancer (antioxidants) and ward off cold and flu viruses (alkaline yielding).

Kale

Kale is one of the best vegetables for you. Kale can ease lung congestion and is beneficial to the stomach, liver and immune system. It contains lutein and zeaxanthin, which protect your eyes from macular degeneration. It also contains indole-3-carbinol, which may protect against colon cancer. Kale is an excellent source of calcium, iron, vitamins A and C, and chlorophyll. Add kale to your "juicing" list and chop it up with your salad greens or in a soup.

Lettuce

Lettuce, like kale, is included in the all-important "leafy greens" category, so it is also a good source of vitamin C, vitamin A, calcium and chlorophyll as long as you are not choosing the iceberg variety. Choose loose leaf romaine, red leaf or other varieties available for you to bag yourself in your produce isle. The lettuce that has been pre-bagged is often washed with a chlorinated solution and should be avoided.

Garlic and Onions

Garlic and onions have both been used in ancient and modern times to treat medical conditions and infections. Because both garlic and onions have antioxidant, anti-inflammatory, antiviral and antimicrobial properties they can also be consumed to prevent viruses. Several of the sulfur compounds in garlic are active against the flu virus.

Some physicians who recommend garlic, suggest taking two garlic capsules a day to treat colds, flu and other viral infections. I prefer fresh garlic to capsules, with the recommendation being to consume at least one and up to twelve cloves per day. Adding fresh garlic to your homemade salad dressing, garlic bread, soups and vegetable juice is an easy way to incorporate more garlic into your diet. Onions, are a close relative to garlic, with similar, though less potent antiviral action.

Onions contain generous amounts of the flavonoid quercetin, which has been shown to protect against cataracts, cardiovascular disease and cancer. In addition, onions contain a variety of other naturally occurring chemicals known as organosulfur compounds that have been linked to lowering blood pressure and cholesterol levels and stimulating the immune system.

Onions contain 25 active compounds that appear to inhibit the growth of cancerous cells with alliin being the main constituent. They have been found to relieve coughs and congestion, especially in the lungs and bronchial tubes. The watery and inflamed eyes due to sinus congestion and hay fever can also be relieved with onion.

Parsley

Parsley is useful as a digestive aid. It also helps purify your blood and stimulate your bowels. Parsley is an anticarcinogen. It contains three times as much vitamin C as oranges, and twice as much iron as spinach. Parsley contains vitamin A and is a good source of copper and manganese. For a natural breath freshener, especially after all of those onions and garlic cloves, chew on a sprig of parsley.

Ginger

Ginger is good for more than just motion sickness and an upset stomach. It also contains ten antiviral compounds. So if you have a viral illness or want to prevent one, drink some ginger tea or add ginger liberally to dishes you cook. Many of the antiviral compounds in ginger also appear in turmeric.

Licorice

Licorice is active against many types of viral infections. One of its eight active antiviral compounds, glycyrrhizin, inhibits a number of processes involved in virus replication. Try drinking a tea made by adding a few teaspoons of chopped, dried licorice root to a cup of boiling water; steep for about ten minutes.

Grapefruit seed extract

Grapefruit seed extract (GSE) is a non-toxic, broad spectrum antimicrobial, antifungal, antiviral and antiparasitic compound prepared in extract form from the seeds, pulp, and white membranes of grapefruit. GSE was developed by Dr. Jacob Harich, a physicist who was interested in studying natural substances that might help protect the body from undesirable microorganisms.

To use the liquid form GSE (it also comes in a powder) to treat viruses, add four to six drops to eight ounces of water or 100 percent juice, stir and drink. It does have a bitter taste, so you may need to plug your nose. It is best to drink this at the first sign of a cold or flu virus, such as that tickling in the back of your throat or the start of clogged sinuses.

Echinacea

Echinacea is by far the most popular antiviral herb. Echinacea fights viruses in two ways. It contains three compounds with specific antiviral activity. Root extracts of echinacea have also been shown to act like interferon, the body's own antiviral compound. In addition, echinacea is an immune stimulant that helps the body defend itself against viral infections.

Go organic if it is on the "dirty dozen" list

The "dirty dozen" list contains the twelve fruits and vegetables most heavily sprayed with pesticides. This list was compiled by the Environmental Working Group from approximately 87,000 studies by the United States Department of Agriculture and the Food and Drug Administration of 47 fruits and vegetables between 2000 and 2007. It is estimated that if you avoid eating the non-organically grown produce on this list, your pesticide exposure can be reduced by up to 80 percent.

Here are the "dirty dozen" listed in decreasing order of pesticide content: Peaches (worst), apples, sweet bell peppers, celery, nectarines, strawberries, cherries, kale, lettuce, grapes, carrots and pears. Additionally, coffee and peanuts should also be organic due to high pesticide exposure.

Buying organic produce is a little more expensive initially, but preventing pesticides, which tax your immune and lymphatic systems, from entering your body is worth it. You will also begin to notice that when you are fueling your body with *real* food that contains live enzymes, phytonutrients, vitamins and minerals, your appetite decreases. This is because you are now nourishing your body's cells and no longer just feeding your mouth with empty calories.

Additional organic recommendations

Dairy products should also be organic. There are three main reasons for choosing organic milk and yogurt. First, you will avoid consuming the pesticides or chemicals the cows consumed when they ate the grass and grains sprayed with pesticides and herbicides. Second, you will avoid consuming any antibiotics or hormones that may have been injected into the cows prior to milking. Third, you will be amazed to notice the improvement in your child's focus and behavior. This last reason is subjective on my part. I have noticed a drastic improvement in the behavior of our children. All three of my children are much more calm, focused and happy since our family switched to all organic milk and yogurt. I am not sure of the reason behind this, I can only speculate.

A bonus benefit is that once you taste how rich and creamy organic milk tastes, you will never want to switch back to your old milk. The one percent milk is so rich, it tastes like two percent milk. When you look for organic yogurt, read the ingredient list to make sure it does not contain corn syrup or artificial sweeteners. Some of you may want to seek out raw milk, which has not been pasteurized from your local farmers. This is a great option for those who are healthy with a strong immune system.

If you are a coffee drinker, at minimum, you should be choosing organic coffee. Due to the high caffeine content, which causes stress to your body, you may want to consider an alternative. Teeccino is an all-natural coffee substitute. It is made from chicory, barley, carob and spices. You brew it just like you would coffee. We like to use half organic coffee mixed with half Teeccino. Their website is www.teeccino.com if you would like to find more information.

Peanuts and peanut butter

When buying peanuts and peanut butter, you should always purchase the organic variety. Non-organic peanuts and peanut butters are very high in pesticides and fungus. They can also contain aflatoxin, a potent carcinogenic (cancer-causing) mold.

Increase alkalinity quickly

If you are under a lot of stress or have been feeling run down, you may be a little on the acidic side, even if you have been working to increase your intake of fruit and vegetables. This will leave your body more vulnerable to the invasion of viruses and bacteria.

If you begin to feel nasal drainage or an itchy throat, you will want to increase your alkalinity quickly. You can do this by adding one-half teaspoon of baking soda to a full glass of water and drinking it. You will want to repeat this for two to three days or until your first signs of a cold or flu subside. You should also plan to "juice" that day (see *juicing*; chapter 8) and sit in a hot sauna to sweat out your acidity and the virus (see *lymphatic system*; chapter 13).

One important point to note: as you begin to increase the alkalinity in your body, you may actually feel as if you have the flu! This is a similar feeling to having an alcohol-induced hangover. This happens because your body needs to get the acid out. You may spike a fever and sweat as your health begins to improve.

This happened to me about half way through the day I was only drinking fresh vegetable and fruit juices. I broke out in a fever and was sure I had the flu for about two hours. This helped me realize the amazing healing powers of fresh juice (see *juicing*; chapter 8).

A friend of mine, at my recommendation, bought some chlorella capsules to assist her in improving her acidic-yielding diet. Chlorella is a single-celled freshwater alga. These algae contain a large amount of chlorophyll, the chemical that gives plants their green color. Chlorophyll is vital for photosynthesis, the process by which plants convert sunlight into chemical energy. Chlorophyll is also available in green leafy vegetables.

Chlorella is beneficial because it binds to toxins, such as heavy metals and escorts them out of your body. When my friend began taking the chlorella, she developed a rash on her stomach and immediately stopped taking them. The rash was most likely her body's reaction to neutralizing the acidity in her body. She gave me the rest of her chlorella and I have been opening a capsule and adding it to my daily smoothie.

Additional oxygen-robbers

Both emotional and physical stress create a very high oxygen loss. Most stress can be either partially or completely managed with aerobic exercise and or proper breathing exercises. See chapter 12 (Immune System) for additional information on managing stress.

CHAPTER 7

Smoothies in the Morning

Our bodies are our gardens—our wills are our gardeners.

—William Shakespeare

Drink your vegetables and fruit.

Smoothies

The easiest way to incorporate more fruit and vegetables into your diet is to consume smoothies. A smoothie is a blender drink that usually has a milk, soy milk, yogurt, fruit juice or water base with fresh or frozen fruit and vegetables added. You can easily add four to six servings of fruit and vegetables to your diet with just one smoothie, which is half of your produce intake goal for the day.

When you first start making smoothies, limit the number of ingredients to three or four. A beginner's smoothie might be one cup of milk, one frozen banana (best if peeled prior to freezing), one-half cup frozen berries or pineapple and a splash of 100 percent fruit juice. Some people may find that adding a few ice cubes helps increase the volume and keep the smoothie cold. Blend this mixture until smooth and enjoy.

As you become more adventurous with your smoothies, you may find that adding a handful of fresh spinach adds a boost of nutrition. A large carrot will add a little color, a bit of sweetness, and the antioxidant vitamin A. Add a tablespoon of flaxseed for some omega-3 fatty acids, texture and healthy vitamins (vitamin E). Don't turn your nose up at any of these suggestions until you try them.

The importance of eating or drinking breakfast

Breakfast is the most important meal of the day. As the word implies, breakfast is "breaking the fast." Unless you eat in the middle of the night, you fast throughout the night. Your metabolism, which is the rate at which your body burns calories, slows during this fasting period. By eating within an hour of when you wake, you break the fast, which tells your body to begin burning calories at a faster rate.

Visualize your metabolism as a campfire. To start a campfire, you start with a small amount of kindling. As the fire starts to burn, you add a little more wood, wait and then enjoy. If you continue to add a little wood, as it burns low, you can enjoy a steady fire all day long. This is very similar to how your metabolism works. If you add a little food in the morning and continue to add more food in small quantities all day long, you will have a steady "fire" burning calories all day long.

Just as you do not throw all of the wood in a pile to start a fire, you do not need a large amount of food to jump-start your metabolism either. This means that you do not need to eat an enormous full-breakfast. Rather, like the small amount of kindling needed to start the fire, only a small amount of food is needed to start your day out right.

The perfect breakfast: smoothies

Make a smoothie in the morning. This smoothie will help jump-start your metabolism and give you a nutritional boost to keep your energy level high all morning long. My favorite blender is the Hamilton Beach personal blender. This is an all-in-one blender in which you can make your smoothie and then put the travel cover on and take with you for your ride to work. You can find it at Target, K-mart or at Target.com for $16.99.

I use this blender at least once daily and it is still running strong after a full year's use. I also enjoy that the cup does not come apart at the bottom, so there is no ring or extra piece to clean. As long as you rinse it out after drinking your smoothie, you will have no problem keeping it clean.

Making a smoothie

You really can't ruin a smoothie. The key is to start with ingredients that you like. If you hate pineapple, you will not want to add pineapple to your smoothie. Start with more fruit and fewer vegetables. Begin to increase the vegetables and decrease the fruit in your smoothie as you can tolerate it.

If your smoothie is too thick, add some more liquid. If your smoothie is too runny, add some frozen fruit or a few ice cubes. If your smoothie is a little bitter or not sweet enough for you, add a splash of 100 percent fruit juice, raw honey or a little Stevia (a natural sweetener) to sweeten it.

If you don't want to add protein powder to your smoothie, but want some extra protein, you can always add a handful of raw nuts or a tablespoon of natural peanut butter to replace the protein you will be missing. While you may taste the protein powder in your smoothie the first few times, you will eventually learn to enjoy it. Be sure to buy protein powder that does not have any artificial sweeteners added, which is most often listed as Sucralose.

Here are a handful of smoothie recipes that you can use to get started. Feel free to tweak the recipes to match your personal tastes and tolerances. After you've made a handful of smoothies, you will no longer need to follow a recipe. All recipes should be blended to desired consistency.

Smoothie Recipes

Basic Good Health Smoothie

1 cup skim or soy milk
1 frozen banana (frozen without the peeling)
1 cup frozen fruit (melon, berries, pineapple)
1 scoop protein powder
a splash of 100 percent fruit juice to sweeten

Advanced Smoothie Recipe (optimal smoothie for weight loss)

1 cup skim or soy milk or water
1 scoop protein powder (whey or soy or pea-isolate)
1 frozen banana (freeze without the peeling)
1 cup frozen berries
1 cup fresh spinach or 1/2 cup loose leaf frozen spinach or other vegetable
1 teaspoon flax oil or 1 tablespoon ground flax seeds
1 teaspoon cinnamon
add a splash of 100 percent fruit juice to sweeten (as needed)

Frosty Pineapple Smoothie (will be thick and sweet)

2 cups fresh cut pineapple
1 cup ice cubes
1 cup vanilla or plain yogurt

Blueberry Orange Dream Smoothie
(orange adds extra texture)

1 cup skim or soy milk
one half medium frozen banana
3/4 cup frozen blueberries
1 whole peeled orange
1 teaspoon flax oil
1 scoop protein powder

Refreshing Watermelon Smoothie

1 cup skim or soy milk
one half medium frozen banana
1 1/2 cup watermelon, removed from the rind
1 cup ice

Berry Protein Smoothie

1 cup almond milk
1 teaspoon vanilla
1 cup frozen cherries or other berries
one half frozen banana
juice of half a lime
2 teaspoons of powdered greens
3 tablespoons whey or soy or pea isolate powder
one half avocado
sweeten with 2 teaspoons agave nectar or 100 percent maple syrup

Refreshing blueberry-lime slushy
(great for afternoon treat)

2 cups ice
1 cup frozen blueberries
1/2 cup purple grape juice
1/4 cup water
1/2 cup seltzer or mineral water
juice of half a lime
1 teaspoon agave nectar or 100 percent maple syrup
garnish with lime wedge

Below is a list of recommended fruits and vegetables that are very compatible with most smoothies. Feel free to experiment with your ingredients to find your favorite combinations and to avoid boredom with too much repetition.

Recommended fruits	**Recommended vegetables**
blueberries	*fresh spinach*
pineapple	*frozen (loose leaf) spinach*
raspberries	*carrots or baby carrots*
strawberries	*cabbage (shredded or wedge)*
blackberries	*avocados*
peaches	*cucumbers*
oranges	
lemons	
limes	

Heart healthy fats

avocado
raw nut butter
organic peanut butter
flax oil or ground flax seeds
raw almonds (soaked in water overnight)

It may sound strange to include vegetables, protein and a fat source in your smoothie. Many of you are used to the Orange Julius version of the smoothie that is a combination of fruit and yogurt. This type of smoothie can get to be quite high in calories and can raise your blood sugar level.

The purpose of adding the protein powder is to keep you feeling satisfied longer and help prevent a spike in blood sugar, followed by a surge of insulin. The flax is added because it contains omega-3 fatty acids that help to reduce inflammation, which can lead to obesity. Adding the vegetables will help dilute the Smoothie's calories and increase it's nutritional punch.

Cinnamon is added because of its ability to stabilize your blood sugar level, raise your metabolism and for added flavor.

When you start making your smoothies, you may want to use a small amount of vegetables and work up to a full two cups of green leafy vegetables. Vegetables will add texture to your smoothie. You may find that using a straw becomes more difficult due to the fiber from the vegetables. Blending longer will help to break the pieces up even finer.

You will notice that adding spinach will make your smoothie turn green. Add blueberries to camouflage the color if it bothers you. The first time I made smoothies with a full two cups of fresh spinach, I told my kids that it would taste minty. They all agreed that it did, including my husband.

If your smoothie is not sweet enough for you, you may want to choose a fruit that is sweeter, such as pineapple. Even canned pineapple comes packed in it's own juice. Save the extra juice and add a splash of this or another 100 percent fruit juice if needed for additional sweetness. Another option is to use vanilla flavored soy milk or add a teaspoon of pure vanilla.

Raw honey, 100 percent maple syrup, and stevia are all natural sweeteners that can be used if you need even more sweetness without sugar. If you currently use artificial sweeteners, you will find that your smoothie is initially not sweet enough. It is to your advantage to begin eliminating all artificial sweeteners from your diet. Soon, your normal threshold for sweetness will return and you will not need to add extra juice or sweeteners.

Chew your smoothies

The addition of vegetables to your smoothie will cause you to need to chew some of your smoothie to break it down further. Even if your smoothie is quite pureed and does not require chewing, you will want to leave each spoonful of smoothie in your mouth for a couple of seconds before swallowing. The reason for this is because your saliva is the first step in the break down of carbohydrates.

Fruit and vegetables are made up of carbohydrates and need to begin the process of digestion in the mouth. You will also be able to absorb more of the vitamins and minerals your body is receiving from the smoothie when you break your carbohydrates down fully. Flatulence, often caused when you increase your intake of fiber in your diet, will also be lessened when you slow down, chew well and leave the smoothie in your mouth longer.

No time to make a morning smoothie?

If you do not have the two or three minutes needed to combine the ingredients for your morning smoothie, you will need to eat something, such as a banana, a handful of Cheerios or a cup of yogurt. Eating on the run is not ideal as a rule, but if you only have a minute or two in the morning, it is far better to eat something instead of skipping breakfast altogether.

If you do not make your smoothie in the morning, you will need to make it at some other time during the day. You may find the solution is to keep your personal blender and smoothie ingredients at work to make during your break. Luckily, it is very easy to clean since it is a one-piece blender unit.

If you just can't tolerate any food in the early morning hours, start with something small, like a few crackers. You only need enough fuel to wake up your digestive system and get your body to begin burning calories. If you have a sensitive stomach in the morning, avoid eating fruit or drinking fruit juice on an empty stomach, as these items may be too acidic for you.

If you think that coffee is the only fuel your body needs in the morning, think again. The caffeine in the coffee will not be effective in getting your metabolism started, and worse, it will fool your body into thinking that it is not hungry. Roughly 30 minutes after you've finished your last cup of java, you will be extremely hungry. Then you will find yourself looking for whatever is most readily available, often the high-fat doughnuts, cookies, or other bakery items that well-meaning coworkers provide.

In the previous scenario, you not only miss out on burning the extra calories that you would have if you had eaten breakfast, but you have also consumed enough fat and calories to smother the fire of your metabolism. The sugary bakery products will also decrease your immune system's virus-fighting potential.

Can I have more than one smoothie a day?

Yes. Some of you will love your smoothie so much that you will want to have a second smoothie later in the day. This is fine. Since your smoothie contains carbohydrate, protein and fat, it is actually a complete meal. If you are craving sweets in the afternoon, the natural sugar found in the Smoothie will satisfy this craving.

Please be aware that if you have not previously been consuming fruit and vegetables on a regular basis, you may want to only start with one per day. This is because your gastrointestinal tract will be a little shocked by the extra fiber you are now consuming and may rebel with excess gas production and sudden bowel changes. After a few weeks of drinking your morning smoothie, your GI-tract should be ready to handle the extra fiber.

CHAPTER 8

"Juicing" Your Vegetables and Fruits

Life is the sum of all your choices.

—Albert Camus

The juice from vegetables and fruit should be called "energy juice."

Juicing for optimal health

A simple way to get the needed vitamins and minerals into your and your kid's bodies is to "juice." This does require a juicing machine, which you can find at Walmart, Target, Kohl's, eBay, and even garage sales. Do the research to find the best juicer for your family. Some of the features you may want to look at include ease of assembly and operation, ease of clean up, the size of the shoot's opening for your fruit and vegetables, and noise level.

I bought my Jack LeLane Power Juicer five years ago when Jack was looking for a spokesperson to promote his juicer in Chicago. When I first started juicing, I had very low expectations and was skeptical. I already regularly made smoothies and didn't know what additional benefits I would get from juicing. As a dietitian, I questioned why you wouldn't want to consume all of that good fiber.

This machine is fairly quiet, easy to assemble, operate, and clean up is minimal. The shoot's opening is large enough to add a whole lemon without cutting it up first. The machine is powerful enough to pull the juice from even the toughest vegetables, as it kicks off a barely moist fibrous pulp on the backside. I often send the pulp through a second time to get the last few drops of juice.

The biggest shock to me was the almost instant surge of energy going through my body after drinking my juiced fruit and vegetables. I felt alert, alive and energized in a strange euphoric new way. The best way for me to describe this feeling is to compare it to the "runner's high" that athletes often experience when exercising. It is so much better than a caffeine-buzz, which I do occasionally enjoy, but is temporary and stressful to your body.

When you are ready to juice your vegetables and fruit, you will want to wash and peel any of your produce that is not organic. You can use a fruit wash such as Fit that you can find in your produce section of your grocery store, but even this will not rid your fruit and vegetables of all of their pesticides.

Clean up is easy when you line the garbage or compost collection side of your juicer with a plastic bag. Once you are finished juicing, you can just toss the bag or take the remnants out to your compose pile. You will also want to fill one side of your sink with soapy water prior to juicing. This is to encourage you to clean your juicer immediately, as the residue will be hard to remove if you do not wash it soon after using.

Yesterday, my nine year old daughter came home from

school and was hungry for a snack. She said she wanted something sweet and was thinking her left over Halloween candy sounded good. I told her she could have a piece of candy if she helped me juice some fruit and vegetables first.

We juiced carrots, apples, celery, parsley and whole lemons. We poured them into pretty wine goblets and sat down to talk about her day. After finishing our juice, she said she was no longer hungry and would wait until dinner to eat again. Her body's cells were hungry and wanted something sweet, but once they were fed with a naturally sweet fruit and vegetable juice, she felt content and did not want the candy.

When you first start juicing, you will want to start with a ratio of two fruits to two vegetables. Ideal fruits for juicing are apples, oranges, grapefruit, pineapple and organic grapes. Ideal juicing vegetables are carrots, cucumbers, celery, kale, parsley and beets. Adding a wedge or two of lemon or lime will cut through the sometimes bitter taste of the vegetables and will also assist your lymphatic system in detoxifying your body.

You want to drink your juice soon after making it, since oxygen interacts with enzymes and phytonutrients in the juice and begins to destroy the nutrients. It is not recommended to juice large quantities to save some for the next week. It is best to consume all of your fresh vegetable and fruit juices within 24 hours to get the most benefit.

Prepared juice that you find in your grocery store has been pasteurized, which deactivates the beneficial digestive enzymes, in order to extend shelf life. Since the enzymes are one of the most important components, giving fresh juices their health-promoting benefit, the bottled juices are far inferior.

When drinking your juice or smoothie, you will want to leave each sip in your mouth for a few seconds to allow your saliva to begin the process of breaking down the carbohydrates into usable energy for your body. This is true of all the food you consume, but is most important for carbohydrate sources.

CHAPTER 9

Salad or Soup at Supper

Enough is as good as a feast.

—English Proverb

Both your waistline and risk of contracting viruses decrease as your intake of vegetables increases.

Plan to consume your largest meal of the day at lunch time. This will give your body plenty of time to digest this meal and will prevent you from feeling out-of-control hungry for dinner. You will therefore, be able to make better choices nutritionally at your evening meal. Do not worry about eating fruit and vegetables at this meal, unless you will not be able to include them at your supper meal. Be sure to include your favorite foods at your lunch meal to prevent feelings of deprivation.

Your goal will be to consume a total of two cups of non-starchy vegetables at your evening meal, which when combined with your morning smoothie, will help you easily reach your goal of 8 to 10 servings of fruit or vegetables per day. The non-starchy vegetables include everything except for corn, peas and white potatoes. These vegetables may be in a big salad, a bowl of vegetable-based soup, steamed, or raw.

Most people will find this volume of vegetables may be enough food for them and they do not need any additional food at this meal. Although this may sound restrictive at first, since you made your noon meal the largest meal of the day, you will not be feeling famished as you sit down to eat your supper meal. Listen to your stomach for the clue as to your hunger and satiety.

Eat soup

Studies have shown that individuals who start their meal with soup eat fewer overall calories at the meal that follows. Soup eaters consumed from 200 to 350 fewer calories than those who didn't eat soup. If you ate soup as an appetizer just two times each week, it would create a calorie deficit that would produce a six to eleven pound weight loss in one year.

Since cream- and cheese-based soups tend to be loaded with saturated fats or trans fats, you will want to limit your intake of these soups unless you have made them from scratch using real ingredients.

Just because soup may be your main entrée at your supper meal, doesn't mean that is all you can have. You may want to add a couple of side dishes, bread or fruit. Your monounsaturated fat may be a little olive oil in the soup, some peanut butter on a slice of bread or a few slices of avocado for a garnish.

Soup can be as easy as opening a can and warming up the contents. The big advantage of canned soups is convenience as well as having the nutrition label so easy to access. You can instantly tell how many calories are in each serving. The main disadvantages of canned soup are that the sodium content is often high and chemicals, such as MSG (mono-sodium glutamate) may have been added. This means that you'll need to drink extra water and avoid weighing yourself the next day because of the potential water weight gain.

Making homemade soup can also be quite simple and quick. A broth or tomato based soup is usually the healthiest choice. Add as many vegetables as you like without any concern about adding excess calories, as vegetables are full of fiber and water with very few calories.

Put your cooked vegetables into a blender and puree to thicken the soup without extra, unnecessary fat. Use lean meat, fish, seafood or skinless chicken breast to add protein without too much extra saturated fat. Any excess fat will float to the top and can be skimmed off once it is chilled.

When ordering soup from a restaurant, remember that the tomato- and broth-based soups will be the healthiest choices, whereas the creamed and cheese soups are much higher in fat content. Be aware of any meat is that is added (sausage contributes the greatest amount of fat).

Salads and the dipping technique

Choosing a salad at your supper meal each day will substantially increase your vegetable consumption. You can load the salad up with vegetables and lean proteins. Be sure to have your salad dressing on the side.

The dipping technique will start to become second nature to you. This is where you dip the tines of your fork into the salad dressing (don't scoop), and then poke your fork into the salad. You will have salad dressing on every bite while only using a fraction of the dressing.

The dipping technique will help you learn to enjoy the taste of your vegetables again. They will not be drowning in dressing, which adds unnecessary fat and calories. Studies have shown that most women get the majority of their fat intake from salad dressings and creamy sauces, which is why women in particular need to be very aware of how much dressing they are using.

Start slowly

You may not like all fruit and all vegetables, but there are so many choices in these two food categories that there must be at least a few you can tolerate. Start eating the few that you do like and then add a few new choices every week. The more fruit and vegetables you eat, the more your body will begin to crave them, and the less your body will crave the less healthy foods.

Begin increasing your intake of fruit and vegetables slowly, because with the extra fiber in these foods, you may experience some bloating and flatulence. The first few days you may just want to add the smoothie. Then add the soup or a small salad for supper. As your body begins to adjust to the extra fiber in your diet, the bloating and flatulence will subside.

You may notice that your bowel movements start to float (in the toilet). This happens because of the increase in fiber and decrease in fat in your diet. This is normal and desirable.

Soup and Vegetable Recipes

Healthy food does not need to be bland and tasteless

Thai Hot and Sour Soup with Shrimp

6 cups chicken broth
3 long strips of lime rind
1 (4 inch) lemongrass stalk, halved and crushed
one half habanero chile pepper, minced
1 cup thinly sliced shiitake mushrooms
1/2 pound large shrimp, peeled and deveined
1/4 cup fresh lime juice
2 teaspoons fish sauce
1 medium tomato, cut into wedges
2 green onions, thinly sliced (1/2 cup)
2 cloves fresh garlic, minced
1 cup light coconut milk
2 tablespoons chopped fresh cilantro

Combine chicken broth, lime rinds, lemongrass and habanero in a large saucepan; bring to a boil. Cook 5 minutes. Add mushrooms and shrimp, cook 3 minutes or until shrimp are done. Add juice, fish sauce, tomato and onions to pan; cook 2 minutes. Remove from heat. Stir in coconut milk and cilantro. Discard lemongrass stalk and lime rinds.

Zucchini-Leek Soup

3 cups chicken broth
5 small zucchini peeled and sliced
1/2 cup sliced leeks, white part only

Combine all ingredients over medium heat and cook until leeks are tender. Cool soup and then place contents into blender and puree. Return to pan and heat to desired temperature. Tell the kids this is "Shriek Soup."

Creamed Soup Mix Base #1

1 cup evaporated skim milk
1 tablespoons cornstarch
1 teaspoon instant bouillon granules

In small saucepan, mix all ingredients together with a wire whisk. Cook and stir until thickened and bubbly. Cook and stir for 1 minute more.

Creamed Soup Mix Base #2

2 cups instant nonfat dry milk powder
3/4 cup cornstarch
1/4 cup instant chicken bouillon
2 tablespoon dried crushed basil
1 teaspoon dried crushed thyme
1/2 teaspoon white pepper

Combine the above ingredients mix and store in an airtight container. Combine 1/3 cup of the mix with 1 1/4 cups of water in saucepan. Cook and stir until thickened. This mix can be sued in place of cream of chicken soup.

Pumpkin Bisque

2 tablespoons olive oil
2 cloves garlic, minced
1 celery rib, diced
1 small onion, diced
1 leek, thinly sliced, white part only
3 cups pumpkin puree (28 oz can)
8 cups chicken broth
2 tablespoon white wine
1/2 teaspoon ground ginger
salt to taste
1/2 teaspoon ground nutmeg
1/2 teaspoon ground cinnamon

Sauté garlic, celery, onion and leek in olive oil over low heat in a soup pot. Cook, stirring occasionally until onion is translucent, 7 to 10 minutes. Add the pumpkin and broth. Bring to a simmer and cook

30 minutes. Stir in the wine and ginger. Season with salt, nutmeg and cinnamon. Serve hot.

Creamy Tomato Basil Soup

3 tablespoons olive oil
1 medium onion, finely chopped
2 pounds ripe tomatoes, roughly chopped
1 garlic clove, roughly chopped
3 cups vegetable stock
2 tablespoons sun-dried tomato paste
2 tablespoons shredded, fresh basil
1 cup milk or almond milk or rice milk
sea salt and freshly ground black pepper
whole basil leaves, to garnish

Sauté onion in oil in a large saucepan over low heat for 5 minutes, stirring, until the onion is softened but not brown. Stir in the chopped tomatoes and garlic; then add the stock and tomato paste. Bring just to a boil, then lower heat, loosely cover the pan and simmer gently for 20 minutes. Stir occasionally to keep tomatoes from sticking to the pan. Transfer the soup to a blender, add shredded basil and blend until smooth. Return soup to pan. Add the milk and heat through, stirring. *Do not allow the soup to boil.* Add additional vegetable stock until you reach the desired consistency. Season with sea salt and pepper to taste. Garnish with fresh basil leaves.

Tomato Basil Soup with Beans

4 cups vegetable stock
2 cups ripe tomatoes, diced
3 cups canned, diced tomatoes
2 cups purple onion, chopped
3 tablespoons garlic, minced
1 tablespoon olive oil
2 tablespoons tomato paste
15 oz can navy beans, rinsed and drained
1/2 cup fresh basil or 2 tablespoons dried basil
1 teaspoon ground white pepper
course sea salt to taste

Sauté onions in large soup pot with olive oil for 5 minutes, add garlic and sauté for additional three minutes. Lower heat slightly and add tomato paste, cooking for a few minutes to caramelize. Add canned tomatoes, navy beans and vegetable broth. Reduce heat and simmer for 25 minutes. Add fresh tomato and cook for additional five minutes on low heat. Pour soup into blender. Process until desired consistency. Add salt, pepper and minced basil. Serve hot.

Creamy Mashed Cauliflower

8 cups bite-size cauliflower florets (1 head)
4 cloves minced garlic
1/3 cup nonfat buttermilk
4 teaspoons olive oil, divided
1 teaspoon butter
1/2 teaspoon salt
fresh ground pepper to taste
snipped fresh chives for garnish

Place cooked cauliflower and garlic in food processor or blender. Add buttermilk, 2 teaspoons oil, butter, salt and pepper. Process until creamy. Transfer to serving bowl. Drizzle with remaining 2 teaspoons oil and garnish with chives. Serve hot.

Broccoli Salad (great substitute for potato salad)

2 pounds of broccoli
1/4 cup purple onion
1/4 cup sunflower seeds or toasted walnuts
1/4 cup Craisins or raisins
1/2 cup olive oil
1/2 cup apple cider vinegar
1/2 cup light real mayonnaise
1/2 teaspoon course sea salt
1/2 teaspoon cinnamon
2 tablespoons raw sugar
1 clove garlic, minced

Combine sugar, cinnamon, oil, vinegar, salt and garlic in a very large mixing bowl. Mix all thoroughly with a wire whisk. Add mayonnaise and mix well. Stir in broccoli, onion, sunflower seeds and Craisins. You can make this as a creamy cole slaw by using half head finely chopped cabbage instead of the broccoli.

Chopped Salad

1/2 box Barilla Plus spiral pasta, cooked
1 head leaf or romaine lettuce, shredded fine
1/2 purple onion chopped fine
1/2 cup shredded carrots
3/4 cup toasted walnuts
1/2 cup blue cheese crumbles
1 clove garlic
1/2 teaspoon sea salt
1/4 cup olive oil
1/4 cup juice from one lemon
1/4 cup plain yogurt or light real mayonnaise

CHAPTER 10

Water and Other Beverage Choices

We never know the worth of water till the well is dry.

—Thomas Fuller,
Gnomologia, 1793

Water is essential for life and optimal health.

Why do I need to drink water?

Water helps you rid your body of toxins, metabolized fat and other waste materials. Your body eliminates toxins with help from your liver, kidneys, intestines, lungs, lymphatic system and skin. Toxins and stored body fat leave your body with urine, bowel movements, breathing and sweat.

Water keeps your skin healthy and resilient. You must replace water frequently, as you lose about two and a half quarts a day. Drinking plenty of water helps minimize sagging skin if your goal is to lose weight. If you are sweating a lot, such as with exercise or visits to your sauna, you will need more water to replace what you have lost.

Muscle contains a large percentage of water. Drinking enough water helps maintain proper muscle tone. Sufficient water intake will also help relieve and prevent constipation. Stools will pass more frequently and without strain if the proper amount of fluid is being consumed. Fiber alone will not cure constipation.

Water is essential for digestion, absorption of vitamins and minerals, circulation, excretion, transporting nutrients, building tissue, and maintaining body temperature.

Older individuals often say they are rarely thirsty. This is because as you get older, your thirst mechanism becomes faulty. You will need to drink water, even though your body may not be sending the signal for thirst. By the time most people become thirsty, they are already slightly dehydrated. Many individuals will eat in relation to thirst, mistaking the signal for thirst as the signal for hunger.

You will find that when you increase your water consumption, your energy level drastically increases. This is especially true if you are currently walking around in a semi-dehydrated state. You may naturally decrease your intake of caffeinated beverages as you increase your intake of water. This helps eliminate the energy surges and drains you may experience in response to caffeine.

Be aware that you will need to frequent the restroom more often as you increase your water intake. Most people only seem to find this an obstacle in the beginning. It could be that they grow accustom to going more often. If you are concerned about waking up in the middle of the night to go to the bathroom, try to finish drinking all of your water prior to 6:00 p.m.

How much water do I need to drink?

Start by drinking eight cups, or 64 ounces, of water each day, as this is the approximate amount you will lose daily. For every

25 pounds of excess weight above your ideal body weight, drink an additional cup of water. If you have 50 pounds to lose, drink 10 cups (80 ounces) of water each day. You can also use the formula of drinking half your weight in ounces daily. Therefore, if you weigh 150 pounds, you should drink 75 ounces per day.

Observe your urine to evaluate if you are drinking enough water. Ideally, your urine should be very pale in color. It should be clear, not cloudy, and without odor midday. Be aware that multivitamins will intensify the color of your urine, as will some fortified cereals, such as Total.

Sixty-four ounces may sound like a lot of water if you are not currently a big water drinker. Once you become accustomed to drinking this volume, you will find that it does get easier. Your body will even start to crave additional water. Those who drink inadequate amounts of water are rarely thirsty. You will find that the more water you drink, the thirstier you will become.

Your body's need for water increases in hot and dry weather, as well as with physical activity. In these situations, it is a good idea to drink some water every 15 to 30 minutes, even if you do not feel thirsty. A healthy adult can survive weeks without food but just a few days without water.

Water retention

For a healthy person who does not have any heart problems or kidney failure, water retention should not be a normal occurrence. If you have a problem with water retention, you will notice that this condition lessens or goes away altogether once your intake of water is up to the body's desired level. Your body retains fluids because it perceives that there is a shortage of water due to inadequate intake. Your body is attempting to hang on to as much of the water as possible to survive.

Your body will go through a period of adjustment as you begin to supply it with the extra water that it needs. Once your body is satisfied that the water shortage is over, it will release the fluid that has been stored in your extremities. You will feel lighter and less water-logged in only a few days. You will also drop several pounds of water weight quickly. If you have retained water in the past, you may come to believe water is the miracle that you've been seeking because it is common to experience a surge in your energy level.

Drink your first cup or two of water first thing in the morning. This helps flush any retained fluids from the previous day and helps increase your thirst for water all day long. Most people find that it is easiest to drink this first glass quickly, even if they are not thirsty, before doing anything else to start their day.

What if I don't like water?

Not everyone will enjoy drinking water. Here are a few tips that may make your new water habit less uncomfortable. Use a straw to help you drink quickly. This is especially helpful if you are having a difficult time consuming the required amount in a day. A large, 32 ounce sports bottle will hold four cups of water, so you only have to drink two full bottles to reach your minimum goal of eight cups of water per day.

You may find it helpful to fill a pitcher with eight cups of water and put it into the refrigerator before going to bed at night. The pitcher should be empty by the end of the next day. If it is not empty, refill it and start over the next day. It will get easier as drinking water becomes a new habit.

Experiment with different water temperatures to determine what you like best. Some research concludes that consuming cold water is best. You will burn more calories because your body attempts to warm it to body temperature. This increase in burned calories is minimal, so don't drink ice-cold water if you prefer tepid. The most important thing is to drink it.

To make your water more enjoyable, try adding lemon or lime wedges or a slice of cucumber. You can also try adding a splash of fruit juice to give it a boost. Avoid substituting other beverages for water. Yes, you are getting some water from your skim milk, fruit juice, or diet soda, but you may also be getting extra calories, chemicals, artificial sweeteners or caffeine too. Aim to drink your full 64-plus ounces of water from actual water and think of your additional fluid sources as a bonus.

Alcohol consumption: Moderation or not at all

Consuming too much alcohol is counterproductive to your goal of preventing cold and flu viruses from making you sick. Alcohol is taxing to your immune system if you drink too much, which can leave your body more susceptible to these viruses.

Alcohol also increases fat storage because of the surge of insulin in the bloodstream following ingestion, slows metabolism and provides excess calories. On an empty stomach, alcohol can increase your appetite as your blood sugar level starts to fall. This is due to your body's response to a surge of insulin.

Finally, a "what the heck" attitude may set in as your inhibitions are lessened with the relaxing effects of the alcohol, which is categorized as a depressant. The best advice is that if you drink alcohol, do so in moderation. Moderation is typically recognized as one drink per day for a woman and no more than two drinks per day for a man.

Diuretic effects of caffeine and alcohol

Drinks that contain caffeine have a diuretic effect on the body, causing the body to excrete more water than it should, which could potentially leave you dehydrated. Not only should you not count caffeinated beverages toward your water intake, but you should also consume more water to compensate for the extra fluids that are pulled from your body. For each cup of coffee you drink, plan to drink an additional cup of water.

Drinking decaffeinated coffee or tea is not the solution. They still contain a small amount of caffeine, as well as tannins. Tannins also act as diuretics to a lesser degree. For every cup of decaffeinated coffee, tea, or caffeinated soda you drink, consume approximately one-half cup of additional water.

Another type of beverage that has a similar but intensified diuretic effect on the body is alcohol. Dehydration and excess acidity are the main reasons individuals experience a hangovers after a night of consuming alcoholic beverages. To prevent this loss of excess body fluids, which causes the headache, alternate each alcoholic drink you consume with a glass of water.

Soda pop

Unfortunately drinking soda pop is not recommended with the *Eat To Beat The Flu* plan. Regular soda contains corn syrup, which is just as detrimental to your immune system as sugar. Diet soda should also be avoided, as the chemicals and artificial sweeteners will create more work for your liver and lymphatic system.

A great alternative to soda is carbonated water or seltzer that you add a splash of 100 percent fruit juice to for flavoring. This is considered a natural soda and will not contain any of the chemicals, preservatives or sweeteners found in regular or diet soda. Most kids find this natural soda to be a real treat.

Green tea, which has been sweetened with stevia, raw honey or 100 percent fruit juice, is an acceptable beverage. Green tea contains antioxidants which neutralize free radicals to prevent cells from turning cancerous. The antioxidant, epigallocatechin gallate (EGCG) found in green tea can also destroy viruses on contact.

CHAPTER 11

Satisfy Your Sweet Tooth Without Sugar

I have a sweet tooth for song and music. This is my Polish sin.

—Pope John Paul II

Sugar is poison to the body and viruses love it.

Some of us avoid sugar because of the calories, others because of the effect on their blood sugar level. Researchers have discovered that consuming refined sugar and high fructose corn syrup can weaken your immune system, leaving you more vulnerable to the invasion of seasonal viruses. I strongly believe removing the sugar from our family's diet during the cold and flu season is one of the most important reasons we are all so resistant to viral infections. You will improve your health by decreasing the amount of or eliminating the sugar in your diet, but only if you don't replace it with something even more detrimental to your health.

Artificial sweeteners are a common substitute for sugar, as

we can see by the large number of individuals purchasing and drinking diet sodas. Unfortunately, the chemicals contained in these artificial sweeteners can have detrimental effects on your brain chemistry and will require your liver to work harder to detoxify your body.

On a personal note, when I was drinking at least six cans of Diet Coke daily, I was in the worst shape of my life. I was overweight, tired, constantly hungry, depressed, my skin was blotchy and my hair and eyes were dull. I am not entirely blaming my poor health during this period of my life on diet soda and artificial sweeteners, but this bad habit certainly was a contributing factor.

Amongst its over 400 jobs, your liver is the organ that is responsible for detoxifying your body of harmful substances. Your liver is also the organ responsible for mobilizing fat from your fat stores to be burned off and used for energy. When you fuel your body with chemicals, toxins (such as nicotine), caffeine, pesticides, artificial sweeteners and overly processed foods, you are overloading your liver and it is not able to perform all of its duties effectively.

One of the best things you can do to keep your immune system strong, to prevent colds and the flu is to replace the sugar and high fructose corn syrup in your diet with better choices. This does not mean that you can never have a can of soda or some sweets. You will just want to avoid them during the cold and flu season or limit your intake.

Nature's candy

You will be pleasantly surprised to learn that your sweet-tooth can easily be satisfied with real fruit. A big bowl of fresh or frozen berries topped with a dollop of organic yogurt is a real treat for your mouth and your body. Berries are sweet, but also contain a substantial amount of fiber which helps keep your blood sugar stable.

The next time you are craving something sweet, eat a fresh fruit first. Then ask yourself if you still want to eat a sweet. Most of the time you will feel satisfied. Sometimes you will want another serving of fruit, but rarely will you still want to eat the refined sugar sweet choice.

Raw honey

Raw honey is a great alternative to sugar for most recipes and to sweeten food or beverages, such as hot cereal or tea. Raw honey contains the live digestive enzyme, Amalyse, which helps breakdown carbohydrates for energy. Once the honey has been heated or pasteurized this live enzyme is destroyed. Raw honey is also antibacterial in nature. My children now prefer honey on their oatmeal instead of brown sugar.

100 percent maple syrup

A great substitute for high fructose corn syrup sweetened pancake syrup is 100 percent maple syrup. You can purchase it by the gallon to make it less expensive. Pour some into a smaller bottle and then freeze the rest to keep it fresh. Its natural sweetness will prevent it from freezing solid.

Agave nectar

Agave nectar is also a super sweet alternative to sugar or pancake syrup. This all-natural nectar comes from the agave plant. It has a low glycemic index, which means that it is slowly absorbed by the body and will not cause the same rapid increase in blood sugar as table sugar. You can use this thick syrup to replace corn syrup in baking and cooking.

Once you begin satisfying your sweet-tooth with more

natural alternatives such as fruit, raw honey, real maple syrup and agave nectar you will start to notice that you are no longer craving process sugar and sweets. Your energy level will rise as you will no longer be experiencing the crashes of low blood sugar levels.

Here is a recipe for muffins where I substituted raw honey for the sugar. I added carrots and apples to boost their sweetness and moisture, as well as their antioxidant and virus-preventing properties. The real bonus is that they taste great and everyone loves them.

Eat to Beat the Flu Muffins

1 cup Hodgson Mill Multi Grain Hot Cereal (not cooked)
1 cup unbleached, all-purpose flour
1 tablespoon baking powder
1/2 teaspoon baking soda
1/2 teaspoon sea salt
1/2 cup raw honey
1 cup shredded carrots
1 cup apples, peeled and chopped
1/2 cup milk
2 eggs
1/4 cup olive oil
1 teaspoon vanilla
1/2 cup pecans or walnuts
1/2 cup 60 percent cocoa chocolate chips

Line 22 muffins cups with paper liners. Lightly spray each liner with canola oil cooking spray. Blend together dry ingredients. Add remaining ingredients and mix until blended. Spoon the thick batter into muffins liners. Bake 12 to 15 minutes or until golden brown.

CHAPTER 12

Strengthen Your Immune System

Life is not merely to be alive, but to be well.
—Marcus Valerius Martial

The key to a healthy immune system is to provide your body with all that it needs daily.

Your immune system

Think of your immune system as an army of millions of microscopic soldiers that operate within you. They go to battle to fight against invading germs to prevent disease within your body. To keep this army operating at peak efficiency, you will want to fuel your body with a diet of high nutritional quality.

Your immune system includes white blood cells, also known as leukocytes, with millions found in each drop of blood to make up approximately one percent of blood volume. Leukocytes defend the body against both infectious disease and foreign materials. They are found throughout your body, including your blood and lymphatic system. An increase in the number of leukocytes over the normal limit is often an indicator of disease.

Another component of your immune system are macrophages, which in Greek means "big eaters." They are white blood cells that are found within your body's tissues. Their role is to engulf and digest cellular debris and pathogens. They also stimulate lymphocytes and other immune cells to respond to pathogens.

The T-lymphocytes are white blood cells that circulate in the blood before migrating to the thymus gland, which is located underneath the top of your breastbone. In the thymus, they develop into specialized helper-T and killer-T cells that are able to identify antigens and infected tissue cells. These T-lymphocytes govern cellular immunity which means they help cells recognize and destroy invading bacteria, virus, and abnormal cell growth such as cancer, and foreign tissue.

Keeping your immune system strong is accomplished by improving your lifestyle choices, such as fueling your body with high quality nutrition choices. Research has found a link between moderate, regular exercise and a strong immune system. You will also want to get plenty of sleep, fresh air, sunshine and pamper yourself with quiet time and meditation.

Enhance your immune system with nutrition

Children and adults who consume diets that are poor in quality will have compromised immune systems and will get sick more often. Strengthening your immune system is as simple as improving your diet by eating more real food. All the antioxidants, vitamin A, vitamin C, vitamin E and selenium (The ACES) are important for immune function. Additional nutrients of importance are also included in this section.

Vitamin A

Vitamin A strengthens the immune system for your nose, airways, throat and lungs. The function of natural killer and helper cells is improved by as little as 30 mg of beta-carotene (converts to vitamin A in your body) per day. This is the amount found in two large carrots. These carrots could easily be thrown into your smoothie, salad or soup.

Vitamin C

Vitamin C is a strong antioxidant that helps your immune system in two of its primary functions to rid the body of foreign invaders and to find any sign of tumor cells. It does this by stimulating the production of white blood cells, primarily neutrophils, which attack foreign substances such as bacteria and viruses. It also boosts the body's production of both antibodies and interferon, the protein that helps protect you from viruses and cancer cells.

The US Recommended Dietary Allowance (RDA) for vitamin C is 75 to 90 mg per day for nonsmokers and 110 to 125 mg per day for smokers. This is the minimum amount which should be consumed for the prevention of disease. For optimal immune function, the goal of 200 mg per day is ideal. Since vitamin C is a water soluble vitamin, excess vitamin C consumed will be excreted in your urine. If you consume too much vitamin C, usually more than 2,000 mg per day, you may get diarrhea.

Meeting this minimum daily vitamin C goal is easy when your consumption of fruit and vegetables is high. Good sources of vitamin C are oranges, grapefruit, lemons, limes, strawberries, cantaloupe, tomatoes, broccoli, bell peppers and leafy greens. One medium orange contains 70 mg of vitamin C and one cup of strawberries has 85 mg vitamin C. Add some strawberries to your oatmeal or some lemons to your water.

Vitamin E

Vitamin E stimulates the production of natural killer cells and enhances the production of the immune cells (B-cells) that produce antibodies. The RDA for vitamin E is 15 mg or 20 IU per day, which is the amount needed for disease prevention. Getting 100 to 140 mg per day, depending on your lifestyle habits, will increase immune function. Those who are sedentary, smoke, drink excess alcohol and have poor nutritional quality diets may require more.

A diet rich in nuts, seeds, vegetable oils and whole grains will help you get vitamin E. One Tablespoon of wheatgerm contains 20 mg vitamin E, one ounce of almonds has 7 mg, one ounce of sunflower seeds has 6 mg and two tablespoons peanut butter has 3 mg vitamin E. Plan to add a few ounces of nuts, seeds or oils to your diet daily to reach your goal intake.

Selenium

Selenium, is a mineral that increases natural killer cells and mobilizes cancer-fighting cells. The best food sources of selenium are fish, shellfish, whole grains, brown rice, Brazil nuts, garlic and sunflower seeds. The RDA for selenium is 55 µg (micrograms) per day. Brazil nuts are unusually high in selenium with just one nut meeting 100 percent of your RDA for selenium.

Vitamin D

Low levels of vitamin D are associated with an increased risk for respiratory infections, such as the common cold and the flu. Scientists from UCLA published a paper confirming two other recent studies, showing that vitamin D is a potent antibiotic. Instead of directly killing bacteria and viruses, this steroid hormone increases your body's production of a class of proteins, called antimicrobial peptides. The 200 known antimicrobial peptides directly and rapidly destroy the cell walls of bacteria, fungi, and viruses, including the influenza virus, and play a key role in keeping the lungs free of infection.

The RDA for vitamin D is 200 to 600 IU, depending on your age. Older people have increased needs. Most of the research that has proven the immune boosting benefits uses 2,000 IU of vitamin D daily. We get vitamin D from food and the sun shining on our skin. Unfortunately we can't get enough sunlight in the winter months. Food sources include fish oil, salmon, mackerel and tuna. One tablespoon of cod liver oil contains 1,360 IU, three ounces salmon contains 794 IU, and three ounces of canned tuna has 155 IU. So, unless you love fish oil, you may need to take a supplement.

If you are concerned about getting the right amount of vitamin D for your body, request your doctor order the 25(OH)D blood test to determine your vitamin D level. Then plan to adjust your diet or supplements based on the results. Remember that you will not need to supplement with vitamin D during the summer months if you get at least 15 minutes of unprotected sun exposure.

Personally, even when supplementing my diet with 5,000 mg of vitamin D daily during the winter months, I still experience seasonal depression, also known as Seasonal Affective Disorder. This is because I live in Wisconsin and cannot get enough sunshine during the winter months. I believe the sun provides us with a mood-enhancing, energizing benefit that is yet unknown. I now spend three weeks each winter in a sunny and warm climate.

Zinc

Zinc is a mineral that increases the production of white blood cells and helps them release more antibodies to fight infection. It also increases killer cells that fight cancer and has been shown to slow the growth of cancer. The RDA for zinc is 8 to 11 mg per day, with 15 to 25 mg per day being a good goal. Be aware that too much zinc (more than 75 mg per day) can slow immune function. Good sources of zinc include oysters, zinc-fortified cereals, crab, beef, turkey, and beans.

Vitamin B complex

The B-complex vitamins are essential to mental and emotional well-being. They help to calm nerves and reduce stress. They also improve blood circulation, therefore enhancing the immune system and lungs. They cannot be stored in our bodies, so we depend entirely on our daily diet to supply them. B vitamins are destroyed by alcohol, refined sugar, nicotine, and caffeine so it is no surprise that many people may be deficient in these.

Some foods which are considered to be high in some of the B vitamins are turkey, liver, liver oil, tuna, chili peppers, lentils, bananas, potatoes, and tempeh (soy based). In addition, molasses and brewer's yeast are good sources of B vitamins. Other meats, dairy products and eggs are high in vitamin B12. Oats, barley, wheat bran, avocado, salmon, Brazil nuts (and other nuts) are more good sources of B vitamins.

Omega-3 fatty acids

Omega-3 fatty acids, found in fatty fish and flax oil, act as immune boosters by increasing the white blood cells that eat up bacteria. An easy way to consume more omega-3 fatty acids is to add one tablespoon ground flax seeds or one teaspoon flax oil to your smoothie daily. My mother used to make me take a tablespoon of cod liver oil when I was sick. I wish she would have known about smoothies!

Tea

Published research from Brigham and Women's Hospital and Harvard University indicates that theanine, an ingredient found naturally in tea, supports the immune system. A cup of tea contains an average of 20 to 25 mg of theanine. Drinking tea throughout the day may strengthen the immune system which is something important to do during the cold and flu season.

Drinking five cups of black tea a day for two to four weeks boosted the body's immune defense system by four times, according to the results of a human clinical trial. According to this study, the data suggests that drinking black tea boosts the body's natural resistance to infection. Tea also contains flavonoids, which are naturally occurring compounds known for their antioxidant properties. Antioxidants work to neutralize free radicals, which scientists believe damage

Eat to Beat the Flu Tea

2 cups water
1 clove of garlic, peeled and crushed
1 inch fresh ginger root, peeled and crushed
1/2 teaspoon cayenne pepper
2 sprigs baby dill
1 bag black tea
juice of 1 lemon
raw honey

Boil the water, and lower to a simmer. Add the garlic, ginger, cayeene, dill, tea and lemon juice. Steep for five minutes. Strain out solids from the tea. Allow to cool for a few minutes and then sweeten with raw honey. Drink both cups. Many people will find that this tea will make them sweat, which helps your body decrease acidity and flush viruses out. This is the ideal tea to drink when you feel a cold or flu starting.

elements in the body, such as genetic material and lipids, and contribute to many chronic diseases.

The CDC states that healthy adults have a 30 percent chance of contracting the flu even with an annual flu vaccination, and the vaccine may be somewhat less effective for children and the elderly. When you are drinking tea in addition to eating more fruit and vegetables and cutting out sugar, it can greatly help your odds of staying healthy.

Eliminate the processed, refined, and junk foods

When you consume the standard American diet, which is filled with processed junk food and sugary beverages, you are creating an acidic, non-oxygenated environment within your body. All viruses thrive in this type of environment. It is best to avoid or limit refined sugars, processed food and fast foods or beverages.

Stress

With our current fast-paced lifestyle, most Americans are faced with elevated levels of stress due to the constant demands placed on them. Some stress is normal and necessary, but the amount of stress placed on us daily is creating an acidic environment that is also weakening our immune system. Exercise, plenty of rest, deep breathing, meditation and a positive attitude can all help control the stress in your life.

Exercise

Lack of exercise or movement can lead to an acidic environment in your body. Ideally, you should move your body for a total of 30 minutes daily. One of the most important reason to get your body moving is for the stress-reduction benefits. Excess stress increases your body's acidity and will cause you to be more susceptible to the invasion of viruses.

Exercise helps increase your intake of oxygen and viruses do not like an oxygenated environment. It also causes you to sweat, which helps to rid your body of toxins and acidity. An additional benefit is that exercise produces endorphins and catecholamines, which help to elevate your mood and control excess stress.

Regular exercise also helps prevent insomnia. Exercising in the early afternoon is the optimal time of day for people who have insomnia. Avoid exercising in the evening because it may increase your alertness and keep you awake.

Importance of sleep to good health

If you are not waking up feeling rested and refreshed, you may be sleep-deprived. The average adult will need seven to eight hours of sleep per night. One of the largest sleep studies ever conducted, on over 12,000 participants found that three important hormones were thrown out of balance with only five and one half hours of sleep for just two consecutive nights.

The three hormones affected are cortisol, ghrelin and leptin. Lack of sleep causes an increase of the stress-hormone cortisol. You will experience an increase in the appetite-stimulating hormone, ghrelin, which increases your cravings for simple carbohydrates and junk food. The third hormone, leptin, is decreased. Leptin acts as your "full-button" sending the signal to your brain telling you to stop eating.

If you are not getting the sleep your body needs nightly, you will have a difficult time improving your nutritional intake. Your appetite will be increased, you will crave junk food and sugary beverages and you will not feel satisfied with a normal amount of food. You will also lack the energy to exercise, which can lead to insomnia the following night.

When your goal is to improve your health, research shows that sleep is as important as eating well and exercise. Research studies have revealed that those who do not get enough sleep tend to have more body fat, partially due to the fact that lack of sleep will increase your appetite. Typically when you have an increased appetite due to inadequate sleep, you are not hungry for fruit and vegetables. Your body craves more calorie-dense foods, such as fatty, fried and fast foods. These calorie heavy foods are an easy way to pack on excess pounds and compromise your health.

To encourage sleep (for those with insomnia), try eating a small, high-carbohydrate snack approximately 45 minutes before going to bed. A few crackers or a cup or two of popcorn is sufficient. The carbohydrates will increase your brain's production of serotonin, a neurotransmitter that causes a calming or sleepy effect on your body. Remember that ideally we would not eat during the two hours prior to going to sleep, but with insomnia, the lack of sleep will be more detrimental to your health than eating a small serving of carbohydrates.

Limit or avoid caffeine and alcohol to promote optimal sleep patterns. Caffeine, being a stimulant, can prevent you from feeling tired when you are. Limit caffeine after early afternoon to prevent this. Alcohol has been found to help individuals initially fall asleep, but then they experience several periods of interrupted sleep throughout the night.

Deep breathing

To take in additional oxygen and promote stress reduction, deep breathing is essential. It is simple to do and can be done almost anywhere. All you need to do is focus on your breaths and breathe deeply for several minutes. Perform this task once or twice daily for a period of approximately seven minutes each time. If you can only do it for a couple of minutes, do it. It is much better than not doing it at all.

There are different deep breathing techniques that you can learn, but do not make this simple activity more complicated than it needs to be. Make sure you are using your stomach muscles during this exercise. Your stomach should expand (inflate) as you inhale and it should go in (deflate) as you exhale. Using your stomach muscles as you practice your deep breathing helps tighten them, which you will be able to see more clearly once you begin losing your excess abdominal fat.

Deep breathing also helps keep you alert because the extra oxygen goes to your brain. This is particularly helpful during a sluggish point in your day. Most people find that practicing their deep breathing techniques is most beneficial in the late afternoon.

Deep breathing is a useful relaxation technique and can be considered a form of meditation. Many people use deep breathing and meditation to help deal with the stress in their lives. You can do your breathing exercises anywhere. Just find a quiet area, close your eyes, and start breathing. Try to avoid letting negative thoughts pop into your head during this time.

One example of a simple breathing technique is called "square breathing." To square breath, you need to take a deep breath in for a count of five. You then hold this breath for a count of five. Next, slowly exhale for a count of five. Finally, hold the breath out for a count of five. Repeat this exercise five to 10 times, or until you begin to feel relaxed.

You may prefer to do your deep breathing exercises while lying down with your eyes closed. Playing quiet music can help create a peaceful setting for this activity as well. With these serene changes, the breathing exercise becomes a form of meditation, which can help lower your blood pressure and improve your mood. So start breathing deeply today, taking in the extra oxygen and enjoy all the wonderful benefits.

Meditation

Meditation is included in the sleep corner of the triangle, as it is a form of rest for both the mind and the body. Meditation helps quiet the mind so that it can focus, which will help your entire body experience a heightened sense of well-being. If you have a lot of stress in your life, you will find that meditation helps bring you back to your inner self by allowing you to let go of the external details of your daily job and life.

Find a quiet place to meditate, where you can calm your mind and totally relax, as you strive to experience inner peace. Close your eyes. Breathe in through your nose slowly and then exhale slowly. A lot of people will find that repeating a mantra word, such as "calm," over and over slowly, will help them feel more centered.

Transcendental Meditation

Over 600 research studies at more than 200 universities, including Harvard, UCLA, and Stanford, have been done on a specific type of meditation called Transcendental Meditation. This meditation has a focus on quieting the mind with breathing and a mantra that is repeated. It is done twice per day for 20 minutes each time.

The Transcendental Meditation (TM) technique settles your mind and body so that your nervous reaction to stress is reduced. TM technique has been found to be the single-most effective program to reduce stress. Other meditation techniques functioned at placebo levels next to TM.

Metabolic waste products are acids (lactic acid, uric acid, etc.), which is one reason why dissolving stress increases the alkalinity of the body. The effectiveness of Transcendental Meditation is evidenced by as 53 percent reduction on overall health care costs and a 55 percent reduction in cancer, as published in the American Journal of Managed Care. For more information about TM, check out their website at www.tm.org.

Emotions, fresh air and laughter

Viruses love angry, worried, hateful people.Your emotions can decrease the overall function of your immune system. The emotions anger, fear, worry and hate all throw poisons into your bloodstream. This compromises the function of both your immune and lymphatic system.

A positive attitude begins with a smile, even when you don't feel like smiling. It is amazing to notice how this simple act can make you feel better. Your smile will also help those around you feel better. Tell yourself and others you are "feeling fantastic" when they ask how you are doing. Soon you will begin to believe yourself.

Researchers at Loma Linda University in California have been studying the effects of laughter on the immune system. Their published studies have shown that laughing lowers blood pressure, reduces stress hormones, increases muscle flexion, and boosts immune function. Immune function is strengthened when laughing raises the level of infection-fighting T-cells, disease fighting proteins and B-cells, which produce antibodies. Laughter also triggers the release of endorphins, the body's natural painkillers, and produces a general sense of wellbeing.

Laughing is aerobic, so it increases the body's ability to use oxygen. Laughter also helps to decrease dopamine levels, which are involved with the stress response "fight or flight." Additionally, 10-minutes of belly laughing gives your stomach the same workout as doing 100 crunches. The biggest benefit of adding laughter to your life is that there are no negative side effects, so give it a try.

Be sure to get outside for at least 15 minutes daily to get fresh air and sunshine. As previously mentioned, you will get vitamin D from the sun shining on your skin, but you will also get some mind-clearing oxygen. It is difficult to be in a bad mood when you are outside experiencing nature. This could be as simple as walking your child to school or taking a 15 minute family walk after school.

As you begin to treat your body well, you will find that you do feel more calm, happy and balanced. Deep breathing and meditation will help calm your anxiety and stress. The little things will no longer bother you, as you begin looking at your life and those you love through new eyes.

CHAPTER 13

The Lymphatic System

Life is like riding a bicycle. To keep your balance, you must keep moving.

—Albert Einstein

The lymphatic system filters out the junk you put into your body.

Love your lymph

Your lymphatic system is like the waste management system for your body. It acts like a secondary circulatory system that lies directly beneath your skin. It consists of lymphatic vessels, nodes and tissue-cleansing lymph fluid. Your lymphatic system is activated when the lymph fluid is pumped. Then the lymph fluid carries your body's metabolic and respiratory waste products, bacteria, toxins, heavy metals, trapped protein and fat globules into the veins of your circulatory system for disposal.

The lymphatic system functions along with the circulatory system in absorbing nutrients from the small intestines. All carbon dioxide and other metabolic waste byproducts travel from each of your billions of cells, carried by lymph fluid. The lymphatic system is basically collecting your body's garbage and disposing of it. The more garbage you put into your body, the harder your lymphatic system has to work.

A build up of waste blocks your cells from receiving optimal oxygen and nutrients, creating the "wet" environment many lymphatic practitioners believe is the single underlying cause of all illness and disease. When your lymphatic system is clogged or overloaded, it will offload the excess waste and toxins it is unable to handle, to the brain and other organs, reducing their ability to do their work. Still more excess will be stored in the fat cells of your body. The excess waste that is stored in fat cells often appears lumpy under the skin, many people refer to these lumpy fat areas as cellulite.

The approach to keeping a healthy lymphatic system is two-pronged. First you should stop putting so much garbage into your body. This includes excessive protein, refined and processed foods, sugar, sweets, caffeine, alcohol, nicotine, red meat and junk food. Dairy foods can also increase lymphatic congestion in some people.

The second prong to optimal lymphatic health is to work with your lymphatic system to help it clear out the waste and toxins. Here are 10 daily choices you can make to help your body's waste removal system:

1. Bounce or jump or swing your arms when you exercise for five to ten minutes daily. Unlike your circulatory system that has your heart to pump it, your lymphatic system does not have a pump. It depends on the contraction of your large muscles to create the pump.
2. Breathe deeply daily for seven to ten minutes. Taking

deep breaths allows you to take in more oxygen, which helps pump the lymph fluid. Exercises that require deep breathing, such as yoga or tai chi, are more beneficial for your lymphatic system.

3. Drink plenty of water. A great goal is 64 ounces of pure water daily. Without adequate water, your lymph fluid cannot flow properly, which will slow down your lymphatic system.
4. Drink diluted 100 percent cranberry juice. Cranberry juice helps digest stagnant lymphatic waste. Dilute the juice at a ration of four to one.
5. Add fresh squeezed lemon and lime juice to your water. The juice from these acidic citrus fruits (produce an alkaline-yield in the body) promote intestinal muscle contractions to speed the elimination of toxins and metabolic waste.
6. Dry brush your skin with a natural bristle brush, prior to getting into the shower. Always brush toward your heart. this stimulates circulation of blood within your body tissues.
7. Get a body massage or give yourself a massage. This manipulates your body's soft tissues (skin, fat and muscle) and connective tissues to improve the circulation of blood and lymph fluid. Massages improve both your circulatory and lymphatic system.
8. Alternate three minutes in a hot shower with 30 seconds in a cold shower and repeat this three times. This helps remove toxins from your skin.
9. Sit in a sauna on a regular basis. Not only is sitting in a sauna deeply relaxing, but it also helps eliminate toxins and acidity through sweating and deep breathing.
10. Fuel your body with fresh, whole, organic real food

and pure water. The enzymes and acids in raw fruit are powerful lymph cleansers, especially when eaten on an empty stomach. Continue to eat more raw fruit, vegetables, smoothies, soups, salads and juices to assist your lymph in keeping you healthy.

Angry, worried, and hateful people

Not only do negative emotions weaken your immune system, but they also cause a dumping of toxins into your lymphatic system. This causes stress on the lymphatic system and increases your vulnerability to cold and flu viruses.

Excess toxins, whether from lymph-clogging foods, stress or anger are stored in your body's fat cells. Picture that dimpling fat area, also known as cellulite, you may have on the back of your thighs. Think of this area as stored toxins.

Saunas

Sitting in a sauna will help you sweat, which helps remove toxins from your body. You will be getting rid of the excess acid that is in your body because of some of your acidic lifestyle choices. Ideally, you would use a sauna on a weekly basis during the cold and flu season. You should also sit in a sauna whenever you feel the first signs of a virus in your body.

After talking to a leading sauna manufacturer in the United States, I learned that whether you use a wet or dry sauna is really a matter of preference. He said that both types of saunas will assist your body in eliminating toxins and acidity through increased body temperature and sweating.

I like to sit in my sauna for five to seven minutes and then rinse off in a cool shower. I then return to the sauna for another three to five minutes, shower and repeat for an additional two to three minutes. In addition to feeling cleansed and lighter after using my sauna, my skin looks great. My face looks like I've just had an expensive facial. I can now confidently go without makeup because of my juicing and sauna habit.

Your local YMCA or fitness center may have a sauna. As saunas gain in popularity, home use saunas are now available at a reasonable price. It is now easy to convert a closet or a corner in your basement to a sauna retreat. Remember to drink plenty of water to rehydrate your body during and after sitting in a sauna.

CHAPTER 14

Preventing Viruses From Entering Your Body

Nature does not hurry, yet everything is accomplished.

—*Lao Tzu*

If only we could put our kids in a protective bubble.

Two points of entry

There are two main points of entry for viruses to get into your body. They are your mouth and your nose. Of course, you already know to wash your hands frequently, especially before eating. You should also keep your hands away from your mouth. This isn't always so easy for kids to do, but constant reminders do help.

When you begin to feel nasal drainage or a sore throat starting, you will want to gargle to help kill the viruses that are entering your body. You can use a commercial antiseptic, such as Lysterine, or warm salt water. Some people may choose to put a teaspoon of baking soda in four ounces of water and gargle this for 30 seconds.

When it comes to your nose, you need to keep it clean. You can easily do this with warm salt water and a Neti pot. Then, you will want to swab your nostrils with a natural oil that will protect these membranes from viruses.

Neti pot

The key is to keep your nose clean and flushed. You may choose to use a Neti pot, which is a small ceramic pot that you fill with warm salt water. You tilt your head to the side and slowly pour the salt water into one of your nostrils and watch while the water drains out of the other nostril. You will want to use the Neti pot on a weekly basis, prior to experiencing clogged sinuses. The purpose of the salt water flush is to keep your nasal passages moist and flush away viral particles before they have a chance to invade your body's mucosa. As an alternative to the Neti pot, you can swab the inside of your nostrils with a warm salt water solution on a cotton swab or use a plastic syringe to flush them.

Travel and school days

When you plan to travel by plane or train, you will want to protect your nose with an oil that is naturally anti-viral and anti-bacterial. My favorite two choices are sesame seed oil and tea tree oil. Both are equally effective, but the sesame seed oil is much less expensive and you can find it in most grocery stores.

Prior to getting to the train station or airport, you will want to dip a cotton swab into the sesame seed oil and swab the inside of your nostrils well to coat them. Repeat this for all family members who will be traveling with you. If you don't have a cotton swab with you, use your little finger and then wash your hands.

Do this same nasal swab with sesame or tea tree oil for your kids who are going to school during cold and flu season. It will offer them protection against viruses entering their nose. This is an all natural preventive measure that can't hurt you, but can only help.

CHAPTER 15

Get Outside and Move Daily

Movement is a medicine for creating change in a person's physical, emotional, and metal states.
—Carol Welch

Fresh air and movement are essential to optimal health.

Get outside

We all need fresh air and some time outside daily, even if it is only for 10 or 15 minutes per day. One of my favorite naturalists is Mike Adams, he is better known as the "Health Ranger" (www.healthranger.com). He questions if many of us aren't suffering from a "nature deficiency." We spend so much time indoors, breathing the recycled air and so little time out in nature. His recommendation is to simply spend more time exposed to the beauty of the natural world.

Even if you live in a cold climate and it is snowing, you surely can handle a short, brisk walk. Lunch breaks usually allow enough time to catch a quick 10 minute walk around the parking lot or block. You don't even need to change into tennis shoes, just start walking.

When you choose to get some movement and fresh air prior to eating a meal or snack, you will be more likely to make better nutritional choices at that meal. The fresh air, along with the feel-good hormones (endorphins) that are released by your body, will also give you an extra boost of energy. This makes taking a walk before eating lunch the ideal time, as many of us feel sluggish as we approach the afternoon hours.

Some of you are thinking of excuses why this will not work for you. There is no excuse for not stepping outside for 10 minutes, whether this is the time of day you choose to exercise or not. Don't stop to talk to anyone or wait for a coworker to get changed into walking clothes; just go.

When you get outside, make a point to breathe deeply to increase your intake of oxygen. Remember that oxygenating your body's cells creates an environment that does not allow viruses, bacteria, fungi or cancer to grow. You will also be taking in additional oxygen when you are practicing your deep breathing exercises.

Aerobic exercise

The word aerobic means "with oxygen." You need to perform exercise during which the body consumes extra oxygen. This includes any activity that elevates your heart rate and increases your rate of breathing. It can be walking, biking, jumping rope, doing fitness videos, or any other aerobic activity that you choose.

Most people are turned off by the word "exercise" because it sounds like hard work. It doesn't have to be. Do you remember what you liked to do as a child? Did you enjoy biking or swimming or doing the hula-hoop? Choose an activity that you enjoyed as a child and try it again as an adult. You will be surprised to find that you may still love this activity. Several of my weight loss clients have discovered that when they ride a bicycle or go for a swim now as adults, they feel like they are kids again.

To get your blood-cleansing lymph fluid pumping, you should choose an exercise that requires you to move your large muscles. Think about the areas where your lymph glands are located, such as your arm pits and the top of your thighs. Excellent choices would be swimming, biking, walking with swinging arms or jogging.

Think of your exercise as moving or "playing" instead of exercising. I like to refer to my exercise sessions as "mama time" because I am taking time to better myself. I've learned that it is okay to take some time for myself, away from my children without guilt. This is called "healthy selfishness," and it is beneficial to our whole family when I return relaxed and happy.

"Healthy selfishness" is when you do something for yourself that takes you temporarily away from others who depend on you. You need to realize that if you don't take care of yourself first, you will not be able to physically or mentally take care of others.

Remember the flight attendant on the airplane telling you that, in the event of an emergency, you should always put your own oxygen mask on before helping your children? This is an example of healthy selfishness. It is acceptable for you to take time for yourself to exercise on a regular basis. You will be an even better care giver once you return.

When to move your body

Morning is the best time for most people to exercise because of their busy schedules. Too many excuses and unplanned events surface later in the day. Your children may have sports or school programs that you need to attend.

You have bills to pay, laundry to do, and a kitchen to clean. Plus a friend may call or stop over to talk or you may just be ready to relax in the evening. Television shows are also much more interesting in the evening than at 6 a.m. Fitness club trainers will tell you that those who exercise in the morning are 90 to 100 percent consistent in their exercise schedules, while those who exercise later in the day are much less regimented.

By exercising in the morning, you only have to take one shower and get ready for the day once. Morning exercisers can roll right out of bed and be ready to exercise in approximately two minutes. If you choose to take the time to brush your teeth and comb your hair it might take a few minutes more. But trust me, no one expects you to be looking your best at six in the morning!

Organize and lay out your clothes and shoes the night before to simplify your morning routine. If you have to dig in the closet for 10 minutes to find your walking shoes in the morning, you will become frustrated and waste precious time. Place your clothes and shoes in the bathroom. When your alarm goes off in the morning, get out of bed and head for the bathroom. You can be fully dressed by the time you stand up from using the facilities.

Never push the snooze button on your alarm clock. It helps to position your alarm clock on the opposite side of the room so that you need to actually get out of your bed to shut it off. Then, don't look back at your bed. Go directly to the bathroom. Looking back seems to magically pull you back into your bed. Also avoid talking to yourself. You will find yourself making promises to exercise later, which never seems to happen.

After you are done with your 30 minutes of activity, you will be very proud of yourself. You will find that you have more energy all morning long, much more energy than if you had slept your precious exercise time away. Your body will also be burning more calories throughout the day.

Exercising later in the day means that you have to tote clothes, hair supplies, and makeup with you to work. It is much more convenient to get your exercise out of the way in the morning. If you do think you will make the time to exercise in the evening, just plan to allow enough time to get cleaned up or shower prior to going to bed.

If you already have an established exercise routine that starts later in the day, that is great and you do not need to change your exercise time. Keep up the good work! Consistency, regardless of the time of the day, is the key.

Frequency and duration of movement

The American College of Sports Medicine and the American Heart Association recommend adults get at least 30 minutes of cardiovascular (or aerobic) exercise, five days per week for optimal health. This frequency and duration of movement will be beneficial in pumping the blood cleansing lymph fluid through your body. Most research agrees that after 60 minutes of exercise, not much additional benefit is added and you substantially increase your risk of injury, so don't over do it.

Schedule your activity into your day as if it were an appointment. Put it in your date book or on your calendar along with your other commitments. Schedule it at a time when you will realistically do it. Scheduling will help you think of your exercise time as non-negotiable. It will also prevent you from scheduling something else during your allotted exercise time.

Don't skip exercise more than two days in a row. The first

day that you don't exercise you will think about it and wish that you had made the time to do it. You will think about the extra energy you had the day before and how good you felt. The second day you skip your exercise session, you will still think about the positive benefits without as much remorse. After skipping your third day of exercise, exercise will become "work" again in your mind. These three skipped sessions can quickly turn into weeks and even months.

Don't think of your exercise time as time lost. Think of it as an investment in yourself. You are much more productive during the rest of your day after getting your blood and lymph fluid pumping, as well as supplying your brain with the extra oxygen it needs for increased concentration.

Set goals

By setting goals, you will keep yourself motivated and constantly working toward something. Your goals may change weekly, such as exercising three times per week for the next four weeks. An excellent method of tracking a goal like this is to hang a calendar in your bathroom or any other location where you will see it several times each day. When you finish your activity, place a sticker on the day or draw a big star with a marker.

At a glance, you will be constantly reminded of how many exercise sessions you have completed each week and month. When the month is over, tally your stickers or stars, write the total on the bottom of the page (such as 19 out of 30), and flip the calendar page to the next month. You start fresh with each new month, but you can look back at your progress anytime.

You will probably start to notice that the stress in your life decreases as the number of stars on your calendar increases. You are not imagining this. Exercise produces natural mood-lifters, called endorphins. They act much in the same way antidepressants do, only without the negative side effects of the drugs.

Some people may choose to set long-range goals, such as participating in an event. This could be a five kilometer walk or even a full marathon or triathlon. Set your goal according to your comfort level and what you wish to achieve.

Isometric toning or "squeezies"

Isometric exercises are when you contract a specific muscle or group of muscles and hold them in the contracted state for a period of time. This could include squeezing your buttocks or gluteal muscles while standing in line at the store. Or holding your stomach muscles tight (pushing your lower back into the back of your seat) every time you are waiting at a red light while in your car. These isometric exercises can be performed anywhere, usually quite inconspicuously to those around you.

Choose the area of your body that you wish was more toned or may be holding stored toxins, such as the cellulite on the back of your thighs. Plan to squeeze these muscles for at least two minutes, twice per day. Stimulating blood flow to this area will also be beneficial at mobilizing body fat and stored toxins. You can also do this by massaging the specific body area you want to improve with or without massage oil. I like to use olive or coconut oil as my massage oil.

CHAPTER 16

Listen to Your Body

If hunger is not the problem, then eating is not the solution.

—Author Unknown

Your body is sending you messages daily. It is telling you what it wants for optimal health.

Are you listening to your body?

Are your listening when your body is talking? Ask yourself what you would do in each of these five different situations. What should you do?

Scenario 1: *You just finished cleaning the garage and your nose feels full of dust. What is your body telling you to do? It probably wants you to flush your nostrils out with some fresh water. Do you do it?*

Scenario 2: *You are raking the lawn and your back is beginning to hurt, but you still have half of the yard to rake? What does your body want you to do? Maybe it is asking* *you to take a break and do some stretches and rehydrate. Do you take a break and stretch?*

Scenario 3: *You have been sitting at your desk, typing away at your computer all day long. Your eyes are starting to cross, you have a cramp in your left shoulder, your neck is stiff and surely your butt must resemble the shape of your chair by now. Your eyes need a rest and you need to get up and move around. Some neck and arm rotations may help get blood flowing again, but what do you do?*

Scenario 4: *You have had a long day and are exhausted, but the dishes and laundry both need to be done. The garbage also needs to be set out tonight, as tomorrow is garbage day. Then you have to bake cookies for the church bake sale and sort through the mail. Sleep will have to wait, you have too much to do.*

Scenario 5: *You are starving. You haven't eaten since dinner last night, but you have to finish that project. You are on a tight deadline and there is no time to waste. Maybe another cup of coffee and a donut will hold you over for now. Your body and your brain both need fuel to keep going. Caffeine and sugar are not the fuel they need.*

Why do we choose to ignore the signals our body sends us? Our body will tell us when it needs a break, needs to stretch, needs some quality fuel and when it is time to take a nap or go to bed. You need to begin to listen to your body and respond to its needs or you will continue to compromise your health.

Eat when hungry and stop when satisfied

Webster's Dictionary describes hunger as "the discomfort, pain, or weakness caused by a need for food." To think of hunger as the need for food helps keep the term fairly objective. We are talking about your body's need for fuel, not your mouth's desire for chocolate or potato chips.

Common descriptions of hunger are "feeling empty," or "feeling like the body needs fuel." The signals that indicate you are hungry include hunger pangs and a growling stomach. Some people may even feel light-headed if they become too hungry, which could be related to low blood sugar levels.

You should eat when you are truly hungry, instead of for a variety of other reasons. When you begin to listen to your body and eat in relation to internal cues, you will be fueling your body for optimal health and energy.

You should be hungry when you start eating, whether you are enjoying a meal or a snack. Eat slowly, chew well and really enjoy the taste of your food while sitting in a relaxed environment. Listen for your "sigh." This is when your stomach has been filled to the point that it is starting to push up on your diaphragm and will cause you to sigh or exhale strongly. This is your cue that your body has received the proper volume of food.

All children are born with a natural sense of hunger and satiety. They request food when they are hungry and refuse food once that hunger has been satisfied. Observe a baby or a toddler to refresh your memory. It is only in our later years that we are taught to eat until we feel uncomfortable. As children, many of us were often rewarded for cleaning our plate with a trip to the zoo or an ice cream cone.

If you have lost your natural desire to eat when you are hungry and to stop eating once your body has been satisfied, you need to relearn this skill. It will take some practice and will initially seem foreign to stop eating when you are no longer hungry, but eventually it will become second nature again.

Does your body want real food or fake food?

Take a good look at the foods you eat on a regular basis. Are the majority of the foods you eat grown with the sun and rain or are most of them produced in a laboratory or processing plant? Think of the real food as "grow" food and the processed food as "fake" food.

Food that has been modified and processed is typically stripped of its healthy qualities and often contains added ingredients or chemicals to increase shelf life. Corn syrup and hydrogenated fats are often added to convenience foods because they are cheap and make the food taste better. There is some question as to whether or not these ingredients are addictive in nature and could be increasing obesity rates.

Eating a diet that consists entirely of real or grow foods is not realistic for most families. Convenience foods do make life a little easier. Make it a point to identify where your food came from at each meal or snack. We may never get to the point where all of our food is coming straight from the farm or out of the garden, but bringing awareness to our food suppliers is the first step.

As you begin to make more real or grow food choices for your body, you will be pleasantly surprised to notice that your cravings for sweets, junk food and fast food start to subside. You will also notice that you are satisfied with a smaller volume of food. This is because your body is now being nourished and no longer needs to send you requests for more nutrients, which are often confused as cravings for junk food.

Carbohydrates

Carbohydrates can be complex or simple. Complex carbohydrates include all fruit, vegetables, legumes, beans, and whole grains. The grains include wheat, rye, oats, barley, and wild rice. Some complex carbohydrates are refined. In the refining process, the bran and germ have been removed and now the gain in no longer a *whole* grain.

Refined carbohydrates include white flour, everything made using white flour (such as white bread, cake, and bakery products), and white rice. Simple carbohydrates include sugar, high fructose corn syrup, honey, candy, regular soda, and other items made using sugar or syrups.

Calories derived from simple carbohydrates are often called "empty calories" because these foods lack essential amino acids, vitamins, and minerals, yet provide a substantial number of calories. As previously mentioned, sugar and corn syrup should be avoided, especially during the cold and flu season. If you do choose to eat or drink simple carbohydrates, please limit your intake to the smallest amount you need to be satisfied. Keep in mind that the less soda, candy, and non-nutritious processed junk food you eat, the less you will crave them.

A diet that is high in simple carbohydrates and processed foods will often produce rebound, low blood sugars. Low blood sugar levels cause intense cravings for even more of these processed foods, such as white bread, potato chips, snack cakes, soda, and other sweets. When you eat too many refined carbohydrates, your blood sugar quickly rises. This causes the pancreas to secrete extra insulin into the bloodstream. The blood sugar levels then drop, increasing the urge to eat even more of the sweets and processed foods.

To break this cycle, which often leads to excessive weight gain, you must decrease your intake of simple carbohydrates and refined foods. The fewer of these items you eat, the less intense your cravings will be. You will experience fewer fluctuations in blood sugars, which will help you feel more in control of your food choices, allowing you to easily improve your diet and your health.

Complex carbohydrates are the preferred energy source over refined and simple carbohydrates. Complex carbohydrates contribute fiber and many essential nutrients, whereas refined grains have been stripped of most of their healthy qualities. The fiber found in the whole grains, fruit and vegetables will help stabilize your blood sugar, lower elevated LDL cholesterol levels, as well as keep you feeling satisfied longer.

When you search for bread or cereals that are a good source of complex carbohydrates and fiber, the word "whole" should be the first word listed on the ingredient list. It may say whole wheat or whole grain on the front of the package, but make sure to check the ingredient list as well. Try several brands until you find one that your family enjoys.

Whole wheat pasta is usually very heavy and chewy. If your family doesn't enjoy this type of pasta, try a whole grained pasta, such as Barilla Plus. This product combines several grains plus some omega-3 fatty acids and is a much lighter and less chewy product.

Protein

Be sure to consume enough protein. Protein intake is necessary for muscle repair. It also helps to keep your appetite under control, preventing hunger cravings, since it delays the rate at which your stomach empties. Protein will help you feel full longer and less likely to want to snack between meals.

Consuming protein will keep you more alert. This is especially important to remember if you have an important project to work on or a meeting in the afternoon, when most people tend to get tired. Include some protein with your lunch meal for optimal alertness.

Women should consume at least six ounces of protein (42 grams) per day and men should consume at least six to nine ounces per day (42 to 63 grams). Each ounce of meat contains seven grams of protein, so if you are reading labels, your goal should be to consume at least 42 grams of protein per day.

Ideally your intake of protein will come from lean protein sources, such as fish, poultry, lean meats, eggs, low-fat dairy, and soy products. Fatty fish, such as salmon, trout and herring are good choices too, as they contain omega-3 fatty acids, which decrease inflammation.

By adding a scoop of protein powder to your smoothie in the morning, you will have consumed 15 to 20 grams of protein, depending on the size of your scoop. You can choose from a variety of protein sources for your protein powder, including whey, soy, hemp or pea isolate. This is an excellent option for vegetarians.

Fat

Your body requires a minimum of 15 grams of fat daily to function properly. This fat is used to lubricate your organs and keep your skin soft and your hair looking shiny. If you are cutting your fat intake too low, you will begin to notice dry skin and hair.

Choose the best fats for your body. In a perfect world, all of the fat sources in your diet would come from fatty fish (salmon, trout, or herring), flax seeds or flax oil, avocados, olives or olive oil, canola oil, raw nuts or nut butters and dark chocolate. All of these fat sources are either monounsaturated fats or omega-3 fatty acids.

Monounsaturated fats have been found to reduce the fat accumulation around the abdomen. Omega-3 fats are associated with decreasing inflammation. These are both desirable qualities for weight loss. Both of these types of fats should be included in your diet daily.

Be aware of where the fat is coming from in your diet. Aim for 90 percent of the fat in your diet to come from omega-3 fatty acids or monounsaturated fats to greatly improve your diet. The fat sources you will want to omit from your diet will include hydrogenated fats, trans fats, saturated fats and fried foods. These are the fat sources that can clog your arteries and can lead to heart disease. Even people who are thin can have clogged arteries.

Know your trigger foods

Most of us know which foods are our "out of control" or "trigger" foods. These are the foods that you feel you cannot stop eating once you start or it triggers an eating binge. This food can be anything from chips with dip to homemade chocolate chip cookies. The specific food is different for each individual. Usually trigger foods are not healthy foods for our bodies.

You will find it beneficial to avoid having your personal trigger foods in your house, especially during the phase where you are actively learning new eating habits. If you feel you can eat just a handful of those Cheetos and be satisfied, plan to sit down at your dining table and eat them mindfully, not while watching television or standing over the kitchen sink. Never eat your trigger food right out of the box or container. Place one portion into a bowl, put the serving bag away and go sit down.

Eating fast food

You may want to limit dining at fast food restaurants because of the limited number of healthy options available. If you do choose to go to a fast food restaurant, it is best to choose a large salad or a sandwich loaded with vegetables. If you do choose to get a burger or fried meat sandwich, skip the soda and French fries or chips.

Prepare snacks in advance

Picture your car's gas tank. Going too long without fueling your car causes it to run out of gas and stop working. Most of us don't like to risk an empty tank in the middle of the road, so we refuel when the gauge first approaches the red "E." Your body is similar in its need for fuel (food). It doesn't operate well without a sufficient supply.

In order to be in control of your food choices, you should eat when you start to notice the first signs of hunger, rather than waiting until you are famished. Prepare by having healthy snacks available, such as cut up carrot and celery sticks and keep your fruit bowl filled.

To prevent your body from becoming over-hungry, you will need to carry some healthy snack options with you. You will then be prepared if you get caught in an unexpected traffic jam or get delayed at work. Without an available snack, you will be so hungry by the time you get home that you may want to dive into a bag of chips like a crazed animal.

Great snack choices should include protein and fiber, both of which will help you feel satisfied longer and prevent blood sugar fluctuations. Examples include:

String cheese + apple
Peanut butter + celery sticks
Carrot sticks + hummus
Hard boiled egg + orange
Cottage cheese + peaches
Pistachios + grapes

As you can see, it is simply a matter of combining a protein source with a fiber source. Some people will make this as simple as packing an extra peanut butter sandwich in their lunch and saving it for snack time.

Some of you will feel perfectly content between meals. Your morning smoothie will probably get you through until lunchtime and if you eat your largest meal at lunch, you may not feel hunger prior to supper. If this is the case, you do not need to eat a snack.

How are you eating?

If you are like the average American who follows the Standard American Diet, you are probably eating too fast. Most of us have heard that it takes 20 minutes for your stomach to relay the message to your brain that you are satisfied and should stop eating. The problem is that it only takes 10 minutes for the average American to eat a meal. This means you could be eating well beyond what your body really needs for energy and tissue repair.

If you are also working on the computer or watching television while you eat, you may not be aware of the physical signals your body is sending you, telling you to stop eating. This is called mindless eating. Mindless eating is responsible for much of the weight gain busy Americans experience.

A great goal is to practice more mindful eating. To do this, take your meal or snack to a table (not your desk) and sit down to eat without any distractions. You will want to chew your food well, eating slow and really tasting your food. See if you can make this meal take a full 20 minutes to eat your meal. Set your kitchen timer to help monitor yourself.

As your stomach fills, it will expand and push up on your diaphragm, causing an audible "sigh". For some people it is a loud exhale, for others just a little "ahhhh". Listen for yours to learn how much volume of food your body really needs. In a perfect world, you would stop eating at this point. This single tip has helped most of my weight loss clients slow down to get more in touch with true hunger and satiety.

Slow down and really taste your food

It is important that you chew your food well and eat slowly. This is much easier to do when you are not over-hungry. When you eat too fast, you don't have the opportunity to really taste your food. The enjoyment in eating happens in your mouth. If you truly want to enjoy your food, learn to keep it in your mouth longer to really savor it. Practice the art of sensuous eating.

Experiment with one chocolate chip. Close your eyes, take a deep breath and put the chocolate into your mouth. Your goal is to see how long you can keep it in your mouth without swallowing it. Most people will be astonished to find out that, when totally focusing on the taste of the food, they are able to make that one chocolate chip last for close to two minutes.

By slowing the pace at which you eat, you will learn to more thoroughly enjoy the taste of your food and will find that you are more satisfied with a smaller volume of food. The secret to being able to eat slow and controlled is to start eating when you first notice the hunger signals, not waiting until you are famished.

Another advantage of slower eating is that chewing your food thoroughly aids your body in digestion. The saliva in your mouth will begin to break your food down into pieces that are more manageable in size for your digestive tract to handle. Your body is able to absorb more of the vitamins and minerals from the food you eat when you chew them well.

Have you ever noticed that a toddler will sometimes have

whole pieces of food in her diaper? This is because she has not yet learned how to chew her food well. It is coming through much the same as it went in.

Sit down and focus

Many overweight people do a lot of "mindless eating." They eat while standing, preparing a meal, driving, reading, or watching television. If you find it difficult to either prepare a meal or clean up after a meal without sampling the food, chew a piece of gum to occupy your mouth so you cannot eat.

Choose a dining area and only eat while sitting in this area. At home your dining area may be the kitchen table, whereas at work your dining area may be the break room. This will take practice and time, but it will help you become much more aware of your food consumption.

Turn off the television and close the magazine. By only eating while you are eating, you will be able to focus your attention on what and how much you are eating. This will help in your effort to slow down, decrease your portion sizes, and listen for your body to give you the signal that it is satisfied.

CHAPTER 17

A New Approach to Eating and Living

It is not the mountain we conquer but ourselves.
—Sir Edmund Hillary

Common sense prevails.

Simple lifestyle choices for virus protection

Congratulations! You have finished reading this book and you are well on your way to reaching your health improvement goals. You will find it difficult to ever go back to your old eating habits and sedentary lifestyle. Your old lifestyle previously left you susceptible to the viruses that cause the flu and colds, despite your numerous hand-washing trips.

For optimal health, you should continue making the same lifestyle choices you have been making during the cold and flu season, all year long. These choices should now be habits and feel more like a way-of-life than a restrictive diet which makes you feel deprived and punished.

Getting started

Getting started begins with your next meal or snack. You can start your healthier way of living today. Don't wait until Monday, or the first day of the month or the first day of the year to get started. There is no time like the present.

What do you need to get started?

1. **A blender to make your daily smoothies.**
   The Hamilton Beach personal blender is the perfect size for individual smoothies and comes with a travel lid. Find it at K-mart, Target or Walmart for $16.99.
2. **Ingredients for your smoothies.**
   Keep plenty of frozen bananas, frozen berries and fresh spinach available for your smoothies.
3. **A juicer to juice fresh fruit and vegetables.**
4. **Vegetables and fruit to make your juice.**
5. **Ingredients to make your salads and soup.**
   Choose your favorite vegetables to add to your salads and soups.
6. **A water bottle made of polyethylene, stainless steel or glass to drink your recommended 64 ounces of water daily.**

The *Eat To Beat The Flu* recommendations are about simplifying your diet as you increase the nutritional quality. You will be learning how to listen to your body and fuel it accordingly. As you begin to nourish your body the way nature intended it to be nourished, here are some of the desire results you will achieve:

- Your blood sugar level will stabilize
- Your lymphatic system will be strengthened
- Your immune system will function at its optimal level
- Your body fluids will return to an alkaline state
- Excess body fat will be burned off
- Your energy level will increase
- You will begin to think more clearly
- You will decrease your risk of contracting infectious viruses
- You will decrease your risk of contracting preventable diseases, such as diabetes, heart disease, stroke, depression, and cancer

A few of the healthy food choices you have added to your diet include fresh juices, smoothies, soups and salads. These food items are all great sources of fiber and water, plus are packed with vitamins and minerals. You are also eating more lean protein and heart healthy fats. Food items you have limited or omitted are foods that are high in saturated, trans and hydrogenated fats, as well as empty calories from sugar and processed foods. More of your food choices are now created in nature than in a factory.

The minimum activity requirements for you and your family members is to get outside for 15 minutes daily and to move your bodies for a total of 30 minutes most days of the week. The fresh air and exercise will both help to reduce stress and strengthen your immune system.

Don't worry if you are not able to follow the *Eat To Beat The Flu* recommendations completely in the beginning. It will take at least a few weeks or a few seasons to establish these new habits. As you build upon this foundation of knowledge and begin adding more healthy habits, you will begin to notice that you are getting fewer colds and are more immune to the flu viruses. Share the simple advice to eat a vegetable-based diet and to avoid sugar during the cold and flu season, with those around you who will benefit from it.

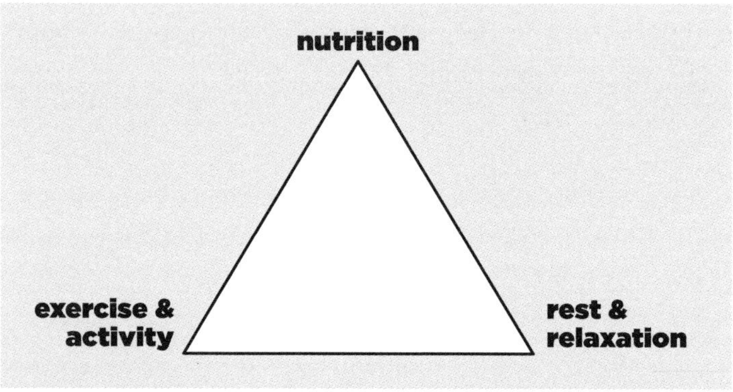

The Wellness Triangle

Remember that the *Eat To Beat The Flu* program is based on the foundation of the wellness triangle. It contains the three equally important corners: nutrition, movement and rest for the body. This triangle represents the ultimate balance for good health in a person's life.

Each corner of the triangle needs to be in balance with the other two corners. When you pay attention to, and begin to make positive changes in all three areas, you will achieve your optimal health goals.

I have simplified your nutrition corner by adding your morning smoothie and your evening meal of soup or a big salad. You are listening to your body and not over or under feeding it. This corner also includes a good intake of water, with limited caffeine and alcohol consumption.

The exercise corner has been enhanced with your 15 minutes of outside time that may also be a period of movement for you. You are also now doing your "squeezies" to tone your body. You should be moving your body for a total of 30 minutes, most days of the week. Being an active person is a bonus calorie-burning and mood-lifting habit.

The rest and relaxation corner of the wellness triangle is optimal when you sleep an average of seven to eight hours each night. You should be practicing stress-reduction techniques, such as deep breathing or meditating daily for at least five to seven minutes. Positive self-talk is also beneficial in reducing stress.

Holidays and vacations

Build as much consistency into your holidays and vacations as possible. When you know that you have a holiday gathering to attend, stick to your usual routine as much as you can, such as getting plenty of sleep, eating breakfast daily and drinking plenty of water. Plan to take a walk for at least 30 minutes on the morning of your event or party. Don't expect perfection and skip the guilt.

Posture matters

The ultimate icing that gives healthy people their enviable position in our society is good posture combined with confidence. When a person walks into a room standing fully erect with their head held high, they possess confidence. We all want to know what their secret is. They automatically appear to "have it all together" with great health and the ideal body.

Practice holding your head high with your shoulders back and walk tall. Pretend that you are royalty when you walk into a room and then observe those around you who are watching your entrance. Smile and act happy, even if you do not feel happy at that moment. Soon you will look and feel as healthy on the outside as you now are on the inside.

What if I return to my old eating habits?

First, stop and take a deep breath. Take a look at what has changed in your lifestyle choices. Why have you started to fall back into your old, unhealthy patterns of eating and inactivity?

Second, take charge of your life again. You only need to remain accountable to yourself. Take out your lifestyle diary or notebook and record everything you put into your mouth. Analyze your intake as if you were a registered dietitian. By now, you know which items may be missing from your diet or which ones are being consumed too frequently.

The third step is to begin recording your exercise sessions on your calendar. This is the best method of tracking your exercise and is quite motivational. Make it a priority to take that 30-minute walk daily and enjoy at least 15 minutes of fresh air during your outside-time.

Fourth, examine your self-talk. Which inner voice are you listening to? You have a little (unhealthy) guy in a red suit on your left shoulder and a thin and an angelic (fit) figure dressed in white on your right shoulder. They are both whispering in your ears. Which one you choose to listen to is up to you. Think about it. Which one is really your friend?

Last, make sure that you are not feeling guilty about the daily choices you make. Focus on what you did do well each day, not on the areas where you may have relaxed your focus for the day. Emphasizing the positive choices will help keep your overall attitude positive.

Visualize your path to improving your health as if it were a road that you are traveling along on a trip to your favorite destination. How long it takes you to reach your destination will determine how many traffic jams and detours you encounter, as well as how many shortcuts you may find. Think of the less healthy choices as the detours that will make your journey a little longer whereas the healthy choices you make are the shortcuts.

The mind is a powerful tool. It has been said, "Where the mind goes, the body will follow." Believe that you are a healthy person who is immune to cold and flu viruses; begin living like this strong and invincible person and soon you will be.

Balance, variety, and moderation

The diet that you choose to follow for the rest of your life needs to be balanced, varied, and likable. You calmly choose foods that are nutritious most of the time and don't feel great guilt over consuming foods that you don't consider "healthy." All foods can fit into your daily diet.

Your attitude will determine your success. You need to love and accept yourself, and praise yourself for your progress. Don't be too hard on yourself if you do make poor nutrition choices or overeat occasionally. It is all a part of the normal eating experience. Trust yourself to balance it out by following your appetite, listening to your body and giving it what it needs and ultimately wants.

SUGGESTED READING

Barone J., Hebert J.R., Reddy M.M. Dietary fat and natural killer cell activity. Am J Clin Nutr. 1989; 50:861-867.

Breathnach, S. B. *Simple Abundance: A daybook of comfort and joy*. New York: Warner Books, 1995.

Collage Video: Exercise and fitness videos. Call 800-433-6769 for a free catalog or visit www.collagevideo.com.

Dove dark chocolate. The inside wrapper contains a positive affirmation; dark chocolate is a good source of anti-oxidants.

Kenfield S.A., Chang S.T., Chan J.M., Diet and lifestyle interventions in active surveillance patients with favorable-risk prostate cancer. Curr Treat Options Oncol. 2007; 8:173-196.

Kornfield, J., S. Salzberg, and S. Young. *Beginner's Mind: 3 classic meditation practices especially for beginners* (audiocassettes). Sounds True Publishing, 1999.

Kratina, K., N. L. King, and D. Hayes. *Moving Away From Diets: New ways to heal eating problems and exercise resistance.* Lake Dallas: Helm Seminars Publishing, 1996.

Lanham S.A. The balance of bone health: tipping the scales in favor of potassium-rich, bicarbonate-rich foods. J. Nurt. 138: 172S-177S, 2008.

Malter M., Schriever G., Eilber U. Natural killer cells, vitamins, and other brood components of vegetarian and omnivorous men. Nutr Cancer. 1989; 12:271-278.

NaturalNews.com

Ornish, D., et al. Intensive lifestyle changes may affect the progression of prostate cancer. J Urol. 2005; 174:1065-1069.

Ornish, D., Magbanua M.J.M., Weidner G., Weinberg V., Kemp C., Green C., Mattie M.D., Marlin R., Simko J., Shinohara K., Haqq C.M., and Carroll P.R. Changes in prostate gene expression in men undergoing an intensive nutrition and lifestyle intervention. The Proceedings of the National Academy of Sciences, 2008.

Pawlak, L. Appetite: the brain body connection. Hermosa Beach: JEBLAR INC., 1995.

Ponichtera, B. J. *Quick and Healthy Cookbook, Volume I: For people who say they don't have time to cook healthy meals.* The Dalles: ScaleDown Publishing, 1994.

Ponichtera, B. J. *Quick and Healthy Cookbook, Volume II: More help for people who say they don't have time to cook healthy meals.* The Dalles: ScaleDown Publishing, 1995.

Redmond L. *Feel Good Naked: 10 no-diet secrets to a fabulous body*. Gloucester: Fair Winds Press, 2002.

Remer T., Manz F. Potential renal acid load of foods and its influence on urine pH. J Am diet Assoc. 1995; 95:791-797.

Rinke, W. J. *Make It a Winning Life: Success strategies for life, love and business.* Rockville: Achievement Publishers, 1992.

Saxe G.A, et al. Potential attenuation of disease progression in recurrent prostate cancer with plant-based diet and stress reduction. Integr Cancer Ther. 2006; 5:206-213.

Seligman, M. *Learned Optimism: How to change your mind and your life* (CD audio book). New York: Simon and Schuster, 2001.

Sell, C. *A Cup of Comfort for Inspiration: Uplifting stories that will brighten your day.* Avon: Adams Media Corporation, 2003.

St. James, E. *Simplify Your Life: 100 ways to slow down and enjoy the things that really matter.* New York: Hyperion, 1994.

St. James, E. *Simplify Your Life with Kids: 100 ways to make family life easier and more fun.* Kansas City: Andrews McMeel Publishing, 1997.

Tolle, E. *The Power of Now: A guide to spiritual enlightenment.* Novato: New World Library, 1999.

USDA Nutrient Database for Standard Reference, Release 12, last updated April 7, 1999.

Warren, R. *The Power to Change Your Life: Exchanging personal mediocrity for spiritual significance.* Grand Rapids: The Encouraging Word, 1998.

World Cancer Research Fund / American Institute for Cancer Research. Food, Nutrition, Physical Activity, and the Prevention of Cancer: a Global Perspective. Washington DC; AICR, 2007.

AUTHOR BIOGRAPHY

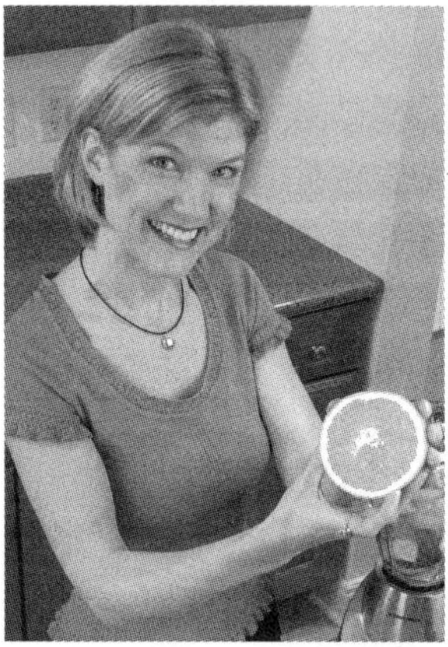

Jill Fleming, MS, RD is a registered dietitian and award-winning health & wellness speaker. She has her masters degree in nutritional sciences from the University of Wisconsin-Stevens Point. She has been teaching audiences the non-diet approach to weight loss and optimal health since 1993. Her first book is ***Thin People Don't Clean Their Plates: Simple Lifestyle Choices for Permanent Weight Loss***.

Jill became passionate about the research behind flu prevention when she realized that her family no longer gets sick with cold and flu viruses. Even though her family of five is constantly exposed to others who are sick, they remain healthy. Their daily food and lifestyle choices were creating an environment, in their bodies, in which viruses could not survive. She wrote this book to help others become resistant to these viruses.

She has been featured in numerous magazines, including *Prevention*, *Family Circle*, *Woman's World*, *Men's Muscle and Fitness*, *Low Carb Energy*, and *Weight Watchers International*. She was even the cover model for *Woman's World* magazine in 2005.

She lives in Wisconsin with her husband and three children. Visit her at www.ThinChoices.com or wwwJillFleming.com. Jill's email is Jill@ThinChoices.com.